EXPLAINING ETHNIC
...FERE..CES

...anging patterns of disadvanta.. in Britain

Edited by David Mason

The POLICY
P~P
PRESS

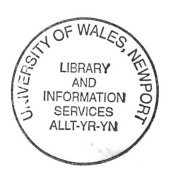

First published in Great Britain in July 2003 by

The Policy Press
Fourth Floor, Beacon House
Queen's Road
Bristol BS8 1PY
UK

Tel +44 (0)117 331 4054
Fax +44 (0)117 331 4093
e-mail tpp-info@bristol.ac.uk
www.policypress.org.uk

British Library Cataloguing in Publication Data
A catalogue record for this book is available from the British Library

ISBN 1 86134 467 8 paperback
A hardcover version of this book is also available

David Mason is Professor of Sociology and Head of the School of Sociology, Politics and Law, University of Plymouth.

Cover design by Qube Design Associates, Bristol.
Front cover: photograph by Peter Marlow supplied by kind permission of Magnum Photos.

Printed and bound in Great Britain by Hobbs the Printers Ltd, Southampton.

Contents

List of figures and tables

Figures

Tables

Foreword

The Cities Programme was set up in 1997 by the Economic and Social Research Council (ESRC) – with the support of the (now) Office of the Deputy Prime Minister – to chart the changing circumstances of UK cities and in particular to explore the relationships between economic competitiveness, social cohesion and governance. It undertook a wide range of studies using different methodologies in many communities, within the UK and in Europe. Much of the work of the Programme can now be found in a variety of academic and more popular publications, including the book of the Programme, City matters (http://cwis.livjm.ac.uk/cities). One important part of the Programme's work was devoted specifically to the role and contribution of different ethnic communities and groups to UK cities and the challenges and opportunities they faced in those cities. For example, our research looked at patterns of education, training and labour market issues, especially for young people, in both the under-performing North and the booming South of England. It explored issues of ethnic entrepreneurship. And it commissioned research on issues of identity, community, citizenship and rights.

The Cities Programme was particularly pleased to support the seminar on which this volume was based. We believed it important to explore in detail the range and diversity of experience of different ethnic groups in different regions in modern Britain. It was obvious to everyone that some groups in some places were doing well. But others were facing persistent discrimination and disadvantage, a fact underlined by the disturbances experienced in a range of northern cities in 2001. This volume was not intended to specifically explore the causes and consequences of those disturbances, although some authors do so. Rather it was intended to look behind those events to identify the nature and sources of the persistent patterns of ethnic and class disadvantage in Britain. The seminar brought together leading researchers in the field with many of the senior policy makers from a range of government departments responsible for shaping and delivering policies in these areas. We were excited by the dialogue that took place on that day. We are equally excited by the prospect of sharing the perspectives and contributions from that day with a wider audience. We look forward to a robust debate about this book's arguments and prescriptions.

Professor Michael Parkinson
Director ESRC Cities Programme
June 2003

Notes on contributors

Malcolm Harrison is Reader in Housing and Social Policy in the Department of Sociology and Social Policy at the University of Leeds. He has published extensively on housing policy, particularly in relation to 'race'. His most recent report (with Deborah Phillips) is *Housing and black and minority ethnic communities: Review of the evidence base* (Office of the Deputy Prime Minister, 2003).

Virinder S. Kalra is a Lecturer in Sociology at the University of Manchester. His main interests are in racism and ethnicity in the fields of employment and popular culture. He is the author of *From textile mills to taxi ranks: Experiences of migration, labour and social change.*

David Mason is Professor of Sociology and Head of the School of Sociology, Politics and Law at the University of Plymouth. He has long-standing research interests in the sociology of race and ethnicity, and he is well known for his work on labour market issues and equal opportunities. Recent work in this field includes research into the recruitment of minority ethnic nurses and on diversity in the UK armed forces. He also has interests in the social organisation of work and the impact of electronic technologies.

Heidi Safia Mirza is Professor of Racial Equality at Middlesex University where she is also Head of the Centre for Racial Equality Studies. She is known internationally for her work on ethnicity, gender and identity in education. Her publications include *Young, female and black* (Routledge), *Black British feminism* (ed) (Routledge) and most recently, with David Gillborn, *Educational inequality: Mapping race, class and gender* (OfSTED).

Tariq Modood is Professor of Sociology, Politics and Public Policy, and the founding Director of the Centre for the Study of Ethnicity and Citizenship, at the University of Bristol.

James Y. Nazroo is Reader in Sociology and Head of the Health and Social Surveys Research Group of the Department of Epidemiology and Public Health, UCL. He is currently joint editor of the journal *Ethnicity and Health*. Ethnic inequalities in health and ethnic differences in health beliefs and behaviours have been a major focus of his research activities.

David Owen is a Senior Research Fellow in the Centre for Research in Ethnic Relations at the University of Warwick. His research interests lie in changing local demography, local labour markets and the analysis of socioeconomic differentials by ethnic group.

ONE

Introduction

David Mason

Background

This volume arises from a seminar entitled *Explaining ethnic differences*, which was jointly organised by the then Department for Transport, Local Government and the Regions (DTLR) and the Economic and Social Research Council's 'Cities' programme[1]. Held in December 2001, the seminar was intended to help inform the policy response to a series of communal disturbances that had taken place in a number of towns, including Bradford, Burnley and Oldham, in the north of England, in the spring and summer of that year. These disturbances, or riots, were notable for the participation of large numbers of young men of South Asian descent, a significant proportion of them Muslim. Such overt conflict between Asian (as against African-Caribbean) young men and the police, was not entirely unprecedented but the scale of the disturbances, together with the involvement of far right white groups, shocked the political establishment and led to series of inquiries and official reports. By bringing together policy makers and social scientists with experience of researching various aspects of ethnic disadvantage, the seminar aimed to explore the current state of knowledge about the structure of ethnic disadvantage and to review explanations for the patterns observed. The chapters that make up this volume are all, with the exception of Chapter Five[2], revised versions of presentations made to the seminar.

Like the report of the Macpherson inquiry into the investigation of the murder of Stephen Lawrence published two years earlier (1999), the urban disturbances of 2001 refocused attention on the continuing significance of ethnic disadvantage for public policy. In this respect, the disturbances might be said to fit into a long-established pattern in the development of policies to address ethnic disadvantage in Britain, that is, the tendency, after a period of public hand wringing and a spate of policy initiatives, for the issue of ethnic inequity to disappear from the agenda for a period, before dramatically being forced back on – not infrequently by events on the streets. In this respect, it might be said that British policy has frequently failed to learn the lessons of the past or, at least, has consistently failed to act on them. Virinder Kalra's contrast between the events following the Brixton riots of 1981 and those of 2001 represents one of the more dramatic examples of the case in point (Chapter

Nine of this volume), but there are others. Thus, there has been a plethora of reports, research studies and good practice guides identifying the key issues that have to be addressed in securing equitable outcomes in recruitment and selection. Nevertheless, it seems that each time a new institution is found wanting, investigations rapidly establish that it has been, wittingly or unwittingly, repeating familiar mistakes, rehearsing familiar excuses, and struggling independently towards solutions, the outlines of which are already well known. Examples include the nursing and midwifery professions (Iganski and Mason, 2002); the police service (Holdaway and Barron, 1997; Macpherson, 1999); universities (Carter et al, 1999); and the armed services (Dandeker and Mason, 2001). Moreover, despite longstanding evidence of the failure of race relations legislation to address adequately the known deficiencies in employment practices, almost a quarter of a century elapsed before the significant strengthening that had long been recommended by the Commission for Racial Equality was introduced.

In some respects, then, the most recent urban disturbances represent a replaying of some old and well-worn themes. At the same time, as reports of subsequent inquiries and investigations have shown (Burnley Task Force, 2001; Cantle, 2001; Denham, 2001), they have also challenged some previously taken-for-granted assumptions about the way policy towards ethnic disadvantage should be framed. In particular, the implications of growing spatial and educational segregation, together with continued labour market exclusion and disadvantage, have raised questions about the effectiveness of some group-centred approaches to policy.

In other respects, the reaction to the 2001 disturbances was more akin to responses to the 1981 Brixton riots (Scarman, 1981) than to the bungled police investigation into the racially motivated murder of Stephen Lawrence (Macpherson, 1999). In the latter case, both Sir William Macpherson's report (1999) and subsequent public commentary focused squarely on the responsibilities of key public agencies, in particular, the police. (This was true also of the heated debate about the concept of institutional racism that followed the publication of the report.) By contrast, the reaction to the events of 2001 replayed themes from an earlier period, including claims of unbridled criminality, the involvement of outside agitators, and suggestions of pre-planning (compare the discussion in Mason, 2000, pp 111-12). In addition, some novel features can also be noted. First, the involvement of significant numbers of young Muslim men fuelled an already emerging process of demonisation, in terms of which young Muslim males began to replace young black men as the object of white fears. These processes had already been given some momentum by the 1991 Gulf War and the Salman Rushdie affair (see also the discussion in Mason, 2000, pp 113, 141-2). They were to be given even greater impetus by the events of September 11.

Second, reports highlighting the significance of spatial and educational segregation for communal relations in the northern towns involved led to the emergence of a new variant of 'victim blaming'. Thus, on the one hand, disadvantaged members of minority ethnic groups were authors of their own misfortune to the extent that they chose to live in close proximity to fellow-ethnics in localities characterised by poor housing and amenities. On the other hand, they were also responsible for the effects of this self-segregation on the community as a whole, undermining opportunities for inter-ethnic interaction and the development of mutual understanding through co-location and education in ethnically mixed schools. As Malcolm Harrison shows, the question of segregation is much more complex than this, arising as it does out of the complex dynamics of the housing system, the distribution of material resources, cultural and religious needs, and a desire for protection from grosser forms of harassment (Chapter Seven of this volume).

In some versions of the voluntary segregation argument, it was even suggested that the real victims, both of minority ethnic residential and educational preferences and of public resource allocation systems, were poorer members of the white community. This was certainly a view put forward by those Far Right political parties that sought to exploit the events. The problem with posing the issue in this way, however, is that it fails to recognise that processes of social exclusion may affect members of every ethnic group – albeit in different ways. While it may well be, as we shall see, that on average members of minority ethnic groups are disadvantaged relative to white people in a range of aspects of contemporary social life, it does not follow from this that all white people are advantaged relative to their minority ethnic co-citizens. Indeed, the 'difference within difference' that Harrison identifies in Chapter Seven is not only a useful term for capturing the way in which experiences of disadvantage vary between minority ethnic groups; it also alerts us to the fact that comparable patterns of diversity are to be found within the white group.

The key to this is to recognise the vitality of class processes in modern Britain. These interpenetrate with ethnicity in a variety of ways in producing and reproducing structures of advantage and disadvantage. One consequence is that it is a mistake to assume, as we all too readily do, that ethnicity is always and inevitably people's primary identity where initial observation suggests that ethnic differences are present and active (see Chapter Two of this volume).

The role of socioeconomic status in providing explanations for differential patterns of ethnic disadvantage is a theme that runs through this book. In addition to their significance for housing, socioeconomic factors play a key role in the explanations for differential health experiences examined by James Nazroo in Chapter Six. The recognition that class continues to loom large in the structuring of opportunities for all groups has also been brought into sharp focus by emerging evidence about the ways in which the experience of disadvantage among different minority ethnic groups is being increasingly differentiated. Nowhere is this clearer than in relation to employment, where there is evidence of upward occupational mobility such that it seems that some groups are increasingly approximating the class structure of the 'white' population, with some even appearing to outstrip white people in their achievements, Chapter Five)[3]. A similar pattern of upward mobility can be discerned in the field of educational participation and achievement, giving some cause for optimism that patterns of occupational mobility might be thereby sustained (Tariq Modood, Chapter Four).

Education highlights another theme that runs through this volume. As Chapters Four and Five both show, there is evidence that minority ethnic students do not receive returns (in terms of labour market success) commensurate with their high investments in education. Similarly, despite evidence of upward occupational mobility, there appears to remain a range of labour market processes that give rise to the kind of continuing ethnic penalty also noted by Harrison (Chapter Seven of his volume). It is difficult to avoid the conclusion that this penalty is a product of continuing processes of discrimination and exclusion. In his discussion of health, James Nazroo comes to a similar conclusion when he considers the evidence that the experience of racism itself may contribute directly to the health status of Britain's minority ethnic citizens (Chapter Six of this volume). The mention of citizenship draws our attention to the particular significance of public policy for people's sense of full, substantive citizenship (Chapter Two of this volume; Mason, 2000, pp 121-35).

While these issues are implicit throughout this volume, they are particularly highlighted by Virinder Kalra's discussion of the criminal justice system and the role of police actions in the disturbances of 2001 (Chapter Nine of this volume). This reminds us that it may well be in the area of citizenship that members of minority ethnic groups are particularly likely to encounter ethnic penalties that have knock-on effects for other aspects of their lives.

This issue of citizenship draws our attention to a crucial dimension of ethnic disadvantage that is frequently overlooked or underplayed. This is the issue of gender. A good deal of literature suggests that gender structures both formal rights and access to full substantive citizenship (see the discussion in Walby, 1994). All too frequently, however, this recognition is lost when attention turns to patterns of ethnic difference and disadvantage. Thus the concept of ethnicity is frequently used as though it were gender neutral, while implicitly – and sometimes explicitly – connoting a male subject. Even when they include a focus on both men and women, discussions of ethnic disadvantage frequently treat women as complicating factors in otherwise gender-neutral analyses. Thus, as Heidi Safia Mirza suggests in Chapter Eight, when minority ethnic women's experiences are thought to follow 'normal' (that is, male) patterns, they are likely to remain invisible in the analysis. When they exhibit distinct gendered patterns, they are treated as analytic exceptions – with subsequent attempts at explanation often entailing processes of pathologisation. Even where they are not disregarded, however, Mirza's analysis suggests that women's agency rarely features prominently. This is because conceptualisations of the agency of minority ethnic citizens, often framed in terms of the concept of resistance, characteristically proceed from quintessentially male public acts – such as the street violence discussed by Kalra (Chapter Nine of this volume). As a result, the less visible acts of mutual support and community involvement undertaken by women are largely overlooked, tending to be seen as features of a private realm traditionally inhabited by women. In the process, the view of some minority ethnic women as passive and subjugated (and hence inevitably invisible) is reinforced, while examples of more assertive public engagement can all too easily be subsumed within the rhetoric of pathology.

The organisation of this volume

This volume is organised around a number of substantive chapters (Chapters Four to Seven, and Chapter Nine) that consider the patterning of ethnic disadvantage in a number of key areas of social life. In each case, the discussion is framed by analyses of continuity and change, with particular emphasis on the persistence of ethnic penalties and evidence of continued discrimination, even in the face of upward mobility. A trio of chapters that provide a range of contextualising information (Chapters Two, Three and Eight) complements these substantive chapters.

Chapter Two seeks to situate the subsequent discussions by providing an overview of the ways in which ethnic difference in Britain has been conceptualised. It argues that experiences of ethnic difference have always been diverse, but that political priorities and analytic practices have frequently masked this diversity. What has come to count as ethnic difference is a product of the distinctive history of postwar migration to Britain from the countries of the former British Empire. As a result, what we can know about those differences – as well as the patterning of change – is to a large extent constrained by inherited categorisation and measurement practices. These in turn may not be wholly consonant with people's own identity choices even though they establish and reproduce a constraining context in which those choices are made. One consequence of this is that the language, concepts and categories used to describe and analyse ethnic difference are highly contested and politicised. Different commentators take different positions on these matters – a fact that will be evident even within the present volume. Moreover, each chapter draws on slightly different data sources. These in turn sometimes utilise ethnic categories that differ from one another. In each case, the discussion has retained the categories found in the original data sources. The reader is referred to these sources for further information and justification of the choices made.

In Chapter Three, David Owen offers an analysis of the demographic characteristics of people from minority ethnic groups in Britain. Like the discussion in Chapter Two, he draws attention to the limitations of the data before going on to provide an overview of the structure of the minority ethnic population. In the process he provides essential up-to-date background information for the discussions in the subsequent chapters of this volume.

Chapter Four, by Tariq Modood, examines the educational experiences of Britain's minority citizens. The chapter examines differences, over time, in the qualification profiles of different minority ethnic groups. It shows that much progress has been made in terms of educational mobility. Modood attributes this to a strong drive for success among most minority groups. Reviewing explanations for continued disparities, he suggests that too much attention may have been given to attempts to uncover the reasons for *under*achievement, while too little has been paid to the reasons for success among those who have made progress.

Changing patterns of ethnic disadvantage in employment are the focus of Chapter Five. The chapter reviews the situation of minority ethnic groups across a range of labour market issues, from participation rates to earnings. It draws attention to continuing high levels of labour market exclusion while also examining the evidence of upward occupational mobility for some groups. These trends are set against the evidence of low levels of household income and high levels of poverty among sections of the minority ethnic population – including some of those apparently experiencing upward social mobility in terms of occupational placement. Reviewing explanations for the patterns observed, the chapter notes the evidence that the investments in education reviewed in Chapter Four do not necessarily attract equivalent returns for all groups. Instead, it is difficult to avoid the conclusion that observable continuing ethnic penalties are linked to the persistence of discriminatory practices.

In Chapter Six, James Nazroo examines the patterning of ethnic inequalities in health in Britain. As with the other chapters in this volume, he highlights the significance of ethnic categorisation and measurement practices for our capacity to produce accurate mapping. In reviewing explanations for inequalities, Nazroo challenges those that draw on crude cultural stereotyping and on simplistic assumptions about genetic difference. Highlighting a theme that recurs throughout this book, he draws attention to the importance of those socioeconomic factors that are, in his view, too readily dismissed in the explanation of ethnic inequalities in health. So, far from being of secondary significance, he suggests that they are probably the crucial element in constructing an adequate explanation. Moreover, he suggests that, in addition to framing access to socioeconomic resources and healthcare services, experiences of racial harassment and discrimination may also lead directly to an increased risk of poor health.

Malcolm Harrison addresses housing in Chapter Seven. He draws attention to the diverse housing experiences of minority ethnic households. Among some minority ethnic groups there are what he calls "many housing success stories". Invoking the concept of 'difference within difference', however, he also shows that there is evidence of continuing patterns of shared disadvantage affecting housing resources, opportunities and choices. Like Nazroo in Chapter Six, Harrison highlights the significance of socioeconomic differentiation for the patterns observed and also shows how factors such as gender and disability may crosscut or reinforce patterns of ethnic inequality. He is particularly concerned to remind us that "negative stereotypes of segregation into so-called 'ghetto' life tell us little about the meanings or shifting characteristics of home and community".

An attempt has been made throughout this volume to ensure that analyses of the patterning of ethnic diversity do not proceed with the assumption that each minority ethnic citizen is a man. Wherever possible, the experiences of women have been addressed and the critical role of gender in shaping and crosscutting ethnic processes has been recognised. Nevertheless, as Heidi Safia Mirza points out in Chapter Eight, too often the very availability of data about women's experiences constrains analysis. In particular, it may lead to what she describes as a pattern of 'normalised absence/pathologised presence' in which women are treated as additional analytic elements, confirming trends already established by looking at men, or regarded as complicating exceptions to 'normal' processes. Chapter Eight is, at one level, a plea for a more central analytic place for women in analyses of ethnic disadvantage and diversity. It represents a claim to analytic resources and for analysts' attention. At another level, however, Mirza is arguing for a reframing of the problematic of ethnic inequality. This reframing demands that minority ethnic groups be treated as active subjects – not in the victim-blaming way explored in Chapters Two, Seven and Nine, but as positive shapers of their own destinies. However, as Mirza points out, it is all too common, when analyses do take account of these processes, for the focus to be on highly visible, public acts. By contrast, she argues that there are myriad ways in which women, in small day-to-day ways, shape their own lives and the futures of their children and communities in a manner that frequently goes unnoticed in conventional analyses.

Finally, in Chapter Nine, Virinder Kalra to some extent changes the focus of the discussion to a, in some ways, more intangible feature of the lives of minority ethnic groups in Britain: the experience of a sense of full, substantive citizenship. A key area in which such a sense has been consistently lacking is relations with the police. Kalra argues that a central issue is the process by which differential ethnic marking of groups takes place in and through the process of policing. Focusing on the civic disturbances that marked a number of England's northern towns in the middle of 2001, he suggests that there are both continuities and changes in the way this process has developed over recent years. In particular, he draws attention to the shift from African-Caribbean to Asian Muslim males as key targets of that marking. Comparing the various official reports of the 2001 disturbances with those of an earlier period, Kalra suggests that a key weakness is a failure to recognise the pivotal role of the police in shaping relations within communities.

Notes

[1] The DTLR has been reorganised since the seminar was held. The responsibility for local government and the regions has since fallen to the Office of the Deputy Prime Minister.

[2] Richard Berthoud of the University of Essex presented a paper on employment at the seminar. Due to other commitments, he was unable to revise it for publication. Consequently, David Mason assumed responsibility for this chapter (Chapter Five of this volume).

[3] At the same time, there are important regional variations in these patterns that are also structured and intersected by the factors of gender, age and religion.

TWO

Changing ethnic disadvantage: an overview

David Mason

Background

In this chapter, I aim to set out the context in which we have to understand the apparent increasing diversity of experiences of disadvantage by Britain's minority ethnic communities. In doing so I shall try, so far as is possible, to avoid anticipating too much of the material that is set out in the following chapters. A key underlying assumption of what I have to say is that neither diversity nor variations in the experience of ethnic disadvantage are new. From the outset, the various groups that have come together to constitute the population of Great Britain have had diverse experiences, both of the process of migration and of establishing their places in an increasingly multi-ethnic Britain. The failure to recognise this diversity probably has a number of sources. These include the initially strikingly visible differences between the newcomers and those already resident in Britain (summed up graphically in the title of Sheila Patterson's book *Dark strangers* [1963]); the adoption for both official and unofficial purposes of the designation 'immigrant'; and a general ignorance about the countries and locations from which migrants had come. Both the general public and policy makers struggled gradually towards a distinction between African-Caribbeans (often referred to as West Indians) and Asians. Only slowly and uncertainly did recognition emerge that the 'Asian' group was not homogeneous, and the significance of different island origins among African-Caribbeans has been all but overlooked.

This is not to say that there are not processes afoot that have made diversity more obvious, nor that there have been no changes in the character and patterning of disadvantage within and between groups[1]. Having said that, the growing consciousness of increasing diversity is a product of a complex of real change, improved data and greater sensitivity to the nuances of ethnic variation. The move away from old assumptions has been greatly facilitated by improved data. Nevertheless, I want to suggest that both past perspectives and the way we are able to grasp the character of current trends are structured by some persistent underlying assumptions about the character of ethnic difference and by our (inherited) categorisation and measurement practices. As a result, even our improved awareness of diversity really only scratches the surface of the real ethnic variety of modern Britain.

Until recently, commentators and policy makers have tended to see ethnic disadvantage as the common experience of an undifferentiated category of 'ethnic minorities' contrasted with the relative advantage of an equally undifferentiated 'white population'. Only slowly and unevenly did recognition emerge that 'ethnic minorities' were differentiated in a variety of ways. Moreover, only in the last 10 years or so has it become common to accept not only that experiences of disadvantage vary but also that some groups appear to be outperforming others on a range of dimensions of social mobility. Even now, however, recognition of that diversity is far from universal, and even those commentators who acknowledge it frequently revert to generalisations about 'ethnic minorities' once lip service has been paid.

Understanding ethnic difference

The reader will have noted that this discussion, indeed the whole book, has been framed in terms of notions of ethnic difference rather than in terms of the concept of 'race'. This reflects the now orthodox position that the concept of race is, at best, an outmoded relic of past scientific error and, at worst, a strategically manipulated ideological category. The arguments surrounding this issue are well known and will not be rehearsed here (see Mason, 2000, pp 5-18, for an introduction to some of the issues). Having said this, it is clear that the terms are widely used interchangeably, in both policy and academic discourses, as well as in everyday speech. Thus, we have policies to counter the 'racial' harassment of 'ethnic minorities' while the term race is enshrined in law itself – in the title and content of the 2000 Race Relations (Amendment) Act. Moreover, even in places where one might anticipate a little more conceptual rigour (such as undergraduate sociology textbooks), the terms are frequently used interchangeably, even when an attempt is made conceptually to distinguish them (see the discussion in Mason, 1996).

In many ways this is a peculiarly British phenomenon. In the US, where the concept of race is perhaps even more entrenched in the national consciousness, as well as in political and administrative life, there is nevertheless a well-established understanding that the concepts are not identical. There are all sorts of intellectual problems with way the distinction is made in the US, but at least it is made. In continental Europe, outside a few Far Right political movements, the concept of race is scarcely encountered at all, other than when incorporated into the term 'racism', which is used generally as a term of disapproval for particular political attitudes and movements.

What, then, are the sources of the persistence of the apparently widespread interchangeability of the concepts of race and ethnicity in Britain? I suggest that they are intimately bound up with the colonial roots of Britain's immigration experience; with the distinctive visibility of those who came to be seen as quintessential 'immigrants'; and with the persistence of a subtext of biological thinking about human difference that, the concept of the 'new racism' notwithstanding, experiences periodic public resurgence (Mason, 1994). As we shall see, this 'racialisation' of ethnic difference (compare Modood in Chapter Four of this volume) is a key to understanding some of the ways in which British conceptions of ethnic diversity have developed.

This is so, despite the fact that the concept of ethnicity represents an attempt to replace an emphasis on physical difference with stress on cultural variation. The late M.G. Smith defined an ethnic unit as "a population whose members believe that in some sense they share common descent and a common cultural heritage or tradition, and who are so regarded by others" (Smith, 1986, p 192). Ethnicity, then, emphasises the social rather than the biological and, importantly, it is rooted at least partly in the self-definitions of people themselves. Much contemporary anthropological and sociological work on ethnicity places emphasis on the processes by which ethnic boundaries are drawn rather than simply reading them off from the existence of apparent cultural difference (Jenkins, 1997). In this view, ethnicity is situational. Whether or not members of a group celebrate cultural markers to distinguish themselves from others depends, in part, on such matters as their immediate objectives, including political and economic ones. This perspective also allows us to recognise that people may have different ethnic identities in different situations. Thus it is possible to be simultaneously English, British and European, stressing these identities more or less strongly in different aspects of daily life. Similarly, the same person might identify him/herself as Gujerati, Indian, Hindu, East African Asian, or British depending the situation, immediate objectives, and the responses and behaviour of others.

The responses of others are important, of course, because they too are making identity choices, and constructing and maintaining their own boundaries. In other words, as well as being potentially situational, ethnicity is also, and fundamentally, relational. Thus no one's choices are unconstrained. This point has a particular significance in a British context since these constraints are nowhere more significant than in relation to public policy and its capacity to frame and shape the opportunity structures in which people play out their lives. In this context, the processes by which ethnic difference is defined and measured play a key role.

In Britain, both in popular parlance and the framing of social policy, ethnic difference is almost exclusively associated with an implicit division of the population into an ethnic 'majority' and a number of ethnic minorities. This distinctive British perspective is substantially a product of the pattern of migration to Britain since the Second World War, a period which has seen the growth of a population whose recent origins lie in the former British colonies of the Indian subcontinent, the Caribbean, Africa, and the so-called Far East. Initially designated in both official and popular parlance as 'immigrants', this population has increasingly become known as 'ethnic minorities'. Two points about this designation are significant.

First, in order to qualify for designation as an ethnic minority, a category of people must exhibit a degree of 'difference' that is regarded as significant. As a result, not every group having a distinctive culture and constituting a minority in the British population is normally included. Thus, the large communities of people of Cypriot, Italian and Polish origin (to name only a few) that are found in many British cities are rarely thought of as constituting ethnic minorities. Similarly, people of Irish descent, a significant proportion of the British population (Mason, 2000, p 21), are rarely so designated. In practice, it is an unstable combination of skin colour and culture that marks off 'ethnic minorities' from the 'majority' population in Britain.

Second, despite the implicit emphasis on difference, 'ethnic minorities' are typically seen to have more in common with one another than with the 'majority'. Diversity *among* the groups so designated is thus downplayed while their purported difference *from the rest* of the population is exaggerated.

Ethnic minorities, then, are those whose skin is not 'white'. There may be differences between them, but these are insignificant relative to their fundamental difference from some presumed British norm – itself marked ultimately by whiteness. One consequence of this is that, as long as priority is assigned by white people to differences of physical appearance, the identity choices of members of minority ethnic communities will be significantly constrained (Modood et al, 1997, pp 295-6).

A further dimension of this problem lies in the distinctive character of British conceptions of ethnicity itself (Mason, 2000, pp 13-14). Characteristically, the term 'ethnic' is taken to refer only to those who are thought of as different from some presumed norm and is frequently used as a synonym for those thought of as culturally different. Talk of an ethnic 'look' in the world of fashion, or of ethnic cuisine, are only two relatively trivial examples of the way white British people are apt to see ethnicity as an attribute only of others – something that distinguishes 'them' from 'us'. Moreover, this apparent denial of their own ethnicity also seems to be associated with a distinctively individualistic world-view in which they see themselves as individuals while others are members of groups. The greater the degree of apparent difference between themselves and others, the more likely British people are to see 'groupishness' as a characteristic of the behaviour and motivations of those others (Dhooge, 1981). One implication of this is that minority ethnic groups can all too easily be seen as the authors of their own misfortunes. In an employment context, for example, a failure to attract applicants from groups conceptualised in this way can be readily attributed to the characteristics of the groups concerned, rather than to the operation of exclusionary processes, or to the rational decision making of individuals. The invoking of parental pressure, or supposed cultural prohibitions or preferences, by some of the respondents in Iganski and Mason's research (2002) may well represent examples of this process at work (see also Chapter Five of this volume). Underlying this process, of course, is a set of scarcely concealed assimilationist assumptions. In the context of the National Health Service, these assumptions have manifested themselves in a variety of guises, including attacks on traditional health practices, the supposedly deleterious health consequences of the 'Asian' diet, scares about tuberculosis, and the relative lack of attention paid to illnesses specific to minority ethnic groups, such as sickle cell disease and thalassaemia[2].

This kind of thinking leads readily to the more or less explicit idea that 'ethnic minorities' themselves constitute a problem. In the context of the earlier discussion of occupational choice, they are a problem because they apparently fail to respond to invitations to join the ranks of professions in which they are underrepresented and which have set themselves the goal of recruiting them. Examples include nursing and midwifery, the police and the armed services (Dandeker and Mason, 2001). Alternatively, they are a problem because they fail to adopt western health practices. Indeed, 'ethnic minorities' have, from the earliest days of postwar migration, been routinely represented as constituting a problem. They were, and remain, a problem for those white people who object to their very presence. They were a problem for governments and others charged with meeting the needs of newly arrived migrants lacking key cultural resources, such as English language skills. They have from time to time been represented as the sources of problems such as certain kinds of street crime.

Measuring ethnic diversity

How ethnic difference is measured exercises a decisive influence over the patterns that can be uncovered. Thus the nature of category systems employed, as well as the purposes for which they were developed, are critical in understanding how ethnic diversity is, and can be, understood. Not only did our current systems develop hand in hand with a particular conception of ethnic difference but, by generating the data in terms of which we can map patterns of ethnic advantage and disadvantage, they serve simultaneously to confirm and reinforce that conception. To the extent that our systems have evolved in the context of a problem–centred view of minority ethnic groups, even if more recently the focus has been as much on the problems faced by such groups, the nature of the currently predominant problem tends to shape the patterns that are uncovered.

The earliest data available on the ethnic diversity of Britain's population relied heavily on an immigration-focused perspective. Until the 1991 Census, the size and shape of the minority population had to be deduced from the place of birth of the head of household (augmented by a number of survey sources). As an ever larger proportion of the minority population came to be born in Britain, this measure became increasingly less reliable as a means of estimating its size. The 1991 Census included an ethnic question, designed to measure the size and make-up of the minority ethnic population. For the first time all members of the population were asked to identify their ethnic group (Coleman and Salt, 1996, pp 9-10). Inevitably, the categories devised for the question were themselves shaped by the patterns known, or thought, to exist.

Thus they proceeded from pre-existing assumptions that had their roots in the beliefs about ethnic difference that I have described and, thus, in earlier conceptions of what problems required to be addressed. Because they inevitably restricted the range of ethnic difference that could be recorded, they contributed to a reinforcement of those assumptions. Even a brief perusal of the relevant question on the Census form illustrates the key point at issue.

Respondents were invited to chose from among the following categories:

White
Black–Caribbean
Black–African
Black–Other (please describe)
Indian
Pakistani
Bangladeshi
Chinese
Any other ethnic group (please describe)

Those who ticked 'white' were not required further to differentiate themselves. It is difficult to escape the conclusion that 'white' was either regarded as a unitary identity or that differences within it were seen as of little importance. At the same time, the other categories represent a curious mishmash of principles of differentiation. Thus they mix, in a variety of inconsistent ways, skin colour, geographical origin, and nationality or citizenship categories. In practice, the only thing that unites them is that they are all presumed to capture the ethnic identities of those members of the population whose skin colour is thought of as not being white. Therefore, the apparent recognition of diversity is immediately undermined by their definition, in practice, by exclusion – they are not white.

The 1991 Census also revealed a further feature of the category systems employed. This is their consistent failure to keep pace with the dynamism of people's self-chosen identities which, evidence suggests, are increasingly volatile and multiplex. Thus, despite extensive pre-testing, the Census results revealed that a significant proportion of those choosing a category other than white were unable to recognise themselves in the pre-coded options on offer and opted instead for self-description. A particular difficulty appears to have been faced by those with mixed origins and those who wished to affirm a hyphenated British identity (see the discussion in Ratcliffe, 1996a). These factors contributed in part to the significant revision of categories for the 2001 Census. This contained a revised question that offered respondents selecting 'white' a further subset of choices. The new categories also permitted greater opportunities for recording mixed origins and for affirming 'hybrid' identities. The Census also introduced a question on religion that, it was hoped, would allow further, fine-tuned, disaggregation of the population.

Nevertheless, it remains the case that underlying the 2001 Census question is still a sense that the most significant ethnic differences are those associated with the conventional British conceptualisation of 'ethnic minorities' described earlier in this chapter; one that is, above all, racialised. The result is that, increasingly sophisticated attempts to disaggregate the minority population notwithstanding, there is still a tendency to conceptualise this population as relatively unchanging both in terms of its boundaries and in terms of the problems to which is thought to be victim. Thus even among those sensitive to equality issues there is a tendency to assume that the problem is to address more sensitively the employment and other needs of categories of people currently recognised as excluded. Those categories, however, are to some degree ossified by the very methods used to identify the patterning of those needs; notably in the Census and other ethnic monitoring categories. The problem, however, is that any such system must always be working with historical data – a problem that is compounded when the categories used for measurement are rooted in historically conceived problems, framed by the gross conceptual distinction between a 'white' majority and 'black' or 'brown' minorities. In other words, it is particularly ill-attuned to keeping pace with changes in the experiences and, crucially, self-identities of those thought to be members of the categories concerned. In addition, the categories have until recently significantly restricted our capacity to measure important emergent differences in the experiences of groups and, even now, they limit the range of the diversity that we can track.

In this context, we should also recognise that ethnicity is not the only – nor even necessarily the most important – component of people's identities. Nor is it always the most significant differentiator in terms of disadvantage. The fourth Policy Studies Institute study, for example, concluded that gender differences are probably stronger and more deeply rooted in the labour market than are those associated with ethnicity (see also Iganski and Payne, 1996). Indeed, as Heidi Mirza shows (Chapter Eight of this volume), gender is a key variable in understanding ethnic differences in modern Britain. In addition, a number of the chapters of this volume also identify the key role of class factors, or socioeconomic status, in shaping life chances.

The irony that he too has been forced to work elsewhere with categories limited in the ways outlined is not lost on the author of this chapter. Indeed, this illustrates the difficulties facing any researcher or policy maker working in this area. They present a fundamental dilemma for the analyst who would be sensitive to the limitations and conditionality of the categories used to track ethnic differences and disadvantage. Any attempt at measurement requires categories. Those categories, moreover, must be capable of tracking changes over time – in other words, there must be some degree of continuity with previous data sources if longitudinal analyses are to be possible. Whatever their limitations, currently available data do provide us with information about real patterns of inequality. What is required is a degree of reflexivity on the part of the researcher to promote that questioning of received knowledge that is the key to making intellectual – and hence practical – progress. Knowing, as we do, that our data tell us only part of the story, we need to be constantly alert to the shifting terrain of inequity and to the dynamic character of both individual and collective identity processes. Post–September 11, we should be particularly sensitive to the ways that events can rapidly and dramatically restructure the ways long-standing loyalties and conflicts are experienced and played out. At the same time, the rapid growth in the population of asylum seekers and refugees, who do not readily fit existing ethnic categories, is having fundamental implications, not only for their own life chances but also for the experiences of long-settled British citizens of minority ethnic descent (conventionally defined).

Ethnic diversity in Britain

We have already noted the extent to which Britain's minority ethnic population is substantially a product of post–Second World War migration. The development of the category 'immigrant' was associated with a view of the already settled population as homogeneous, and having a primordial cultural and national unity. What this perspective failed to acknowledge, however, was that migrations of populations are probably as old as human kind. Certainly if, as is commonly supposed, the human species has its origins in Africa, its migration from its place of origin was a necessary condition for the colonisation of almost every corner of the planet by members of our species. In more recent times, what we think of today as the population of England has been a product of successive migrations and conquests including those associated with the Romans, Vikings and Normans. Indeed, it is noteworthy that a concept often invoked to express a sense of long-standing, or primordial, *English* identity is the term Anglo-Saxon – a concept that itself embodies an admixture of two distinct peoples of Teutonic origin. Interestingly, it appears that this sense of primordial unity is historically quite specific. For example, as recently as 1867, *The Times* noted:

> there is hardly such a thing as a pure Englishman in this island. In place of the rather vulgarised and very inaccurate phrase, Anglo-Saxon, our national denomination, to be strictly correct, would be a composite of a dozen national titles. (Quoted in Walvin, 1984, p 19)

In addition, Colin Kidd (1999) has argued that, in the 17th century, there were at least eight versions of the English story – all of them related to different political projects ranging from Royalism to Leveller radicalism. A common problem for all of them was how to weave the diverse histories of the various groups out of which England had emerged, into a coherent national story. Similarly, Linda Colley has shown in her major study *Britons* (1992) that the *British* nation was invented in the wake of the 1707 Act of Union. It was forged as a national identity in and through a series of conflicts, notably with France, over a period of about a century and a half. So successful was this process that, until brought into question by recent developments, the existence of a British national identity was rarely, if ever, challenged. Yet it was quintessentially a political project in which a new set of ethnic boundaries was consciously erected and celebrated.

Ethnic diversity, then, is not a new phenomenon in these islands. Even in the period now commonly associated with mass migration – the post Second World War period – those entering Britain were diverse in a range of ways. Moreover, only some of them – those with black or brown skins – came to be labelled as ethnically different. Even among these groups, there were huge, if frequently unrecognised, differences associated, inter alia, with geographical origin, religion, language, date of arrival, cultural and financial capital, gender mix and place of settlement (see Chapter Three of this volume). Their largely common experience of downward occupational mobility varied in kind and degree, while they were differentially excluded and incorporated in aspects of social life ranging from the dance hall to the housing market.

Housing, indeed, has been a key strain point at various times in the postwar period. Much of the early opposition to 'immigration' centred on conflicts over housing – a process exacerbated by the serious shortage of accommodation well into the 1970s. More recently, civil disturbances in a number of northern towns in 2001 appear to have been related to emergent patterns of ethnic residential segregation, although as both Chapters Seven and Nine in this volume show, neither the patterns nor their relationship to conflict are straightforward.

Despite the manifest diversity of Britain's new citizens, it is clear that only slowly did our recognition and understanding of differences develop. In the first instance, this took the form of a crude dualism distinguishing 'Asians' from those of Caribbean origin. That early distinction probably owed much to the continuing heritage of race thinking to which I referred earlier. It also had its roots in the political divisions of empire, themselves not uninformed by racial ideologies, in the distinctive arrangements by which different parts of empire were governed and, crucially, in the heritage of slavery.

More recently, the availability of data revealing differential rates of occupational and social mobility (see Chapter Five of this volume) has permitted a more sophisticated and fine-tuned understanding of the diversity of Britain's minority ethnic population, as well as the complex patterning of disadvantage. Past failures of understanding, however, should caution us against assuming that we now have a complete grasp of the ethnic diversity that is modern Britain. The continuing dynamism of ethnic identities, operating hand in hand with emergent structural processes, means that we are continually seeking to capture the essence of what is an ever-changing picture.

It may well be that it is in the area of shifting identities that some of the key processes that will shape Britain's experience over the next century are to be found. Certainly, there are processes afoot that are increasingly challenging many of the things we have come to take for granted about ethnic – and for that matter, national – identities. One does not need to subscribe to the 'breakup of Britain' thesis (Nairn, 1981) to recognise that the process of devolution has led to a reinvigoration of long-standing national identities among both the Scots and the Welsh. Hand in hand with devolution is a growing regional agenda, at both national and EU levels, that has the potential to reawaken regional identities that have long appeared dormant. An interesting by-product of these developments has been the way in which Englishness as an identity has been increasingly problematised (McCrone and Kiely, 2000). As the dominant national group in Britain, it was not necessary until recently for most English people to reflect upon the relationship between English and British identities. With the increasing assertiveness of other national identities within Britain, however, the English are being forced to confront the question of what exactly marks them off. This has been reflected in a flurry of recent television programmes and press commentary asking 'who are the English?' (for example, Paxman, 1999). At the same time, the identities of those whose place once appeared fixed – the so-called ethnic minorities – are themselves undergoing complex and fundamental changes. Of particular note are increasingly common hybrid identities, such as Black-British and Pakistani-British, which challenge still further what was until recently an apparently unproblematic national category (Modood, 1997c).

Ethnic diversity, disadvantage and citizenship

As Chapters Four and Five of this volume make clear, hand in hand with changing identities are a number of structural changes in patterns of educational and labour market placement. As these chapters show, the patterns are complex and it is constantly necessary to remember that evidence of upward mobility for some is not incompatible with continued disadvantage, discrimination and exclusion. Even among those apparently benefiting from upward occupational mobility, patterns of exclusion – or conditional inclusion – are clearly evident. Indeed, it appears that, in some key respects, the message is one that records burgeoning achievement *despite* continued discrimination. Moreover, there is no straightforward relationship between upward mobility and improved material well-being.

At the same time, there is continued evidence that Britain's minority ethnic citizens continue to experience a sense of exclusion from full, substantive citizenship. Examples include: the effects of increasingly restrictive citizenship and immigration legislation (itself exacerbated by recent political controversies surrounding asylum seekers and refugees); arrangements for access to social services and healthcare; and a sense of incomplete incorporation into national political institutions (Mason, 2000, pp 121-35). Perhaps the key area in which this lack of full citizenship has been felt is that of the criminal justice system – and particularly relations with the police. In the wake of the murder of Stephen Lawrence and the subsequent inquiry into the police investigation, much attention has focused on efforts to rid the police, and other institutions, of what is now widely understood as institutional racism.

Against this background, we should note the extent to which, not for the first time, the urban disorders of 2001 highlighted the consequences of social exclusion in this widest sense (compare Jewson, 1990). Although much of the subsequent commentary has stressed the significance of patterns of community settlement and segregation (see Chapter Seven of this volume), Virinder Kalra in this volume stresses the extent to which, just as in 1981, police tactics and relations with the communities concerned played a key part in events as they unfolded (Chapter Nine). The 2001 disturbances also illustrated how, in many deprived areas, the 'white' population also frequently experiences exclusion, albeit differently mediated and labelled. This can all too easily fuel damaging inter-ethnic conflict, particularly when it is exploited by Far Right political parties. Once again, this points to the dangers of conceiving ethnic difference in a way that fails to recognise the diversity of the 'white' population or that aspects of their experience may be shared with those who are ostensibly ethnically different. Again, understanding the ways in which class and gender intersect with ethnic differences is a key to beginning to unravel the complexities involved.

The key message of this chapter, as indeed of the volume as a whole, is that diversity is endemic, dynamic and multi-faceted. It is endemic, not simply empirically, but also because it is intrinsic to the very concept of ethnicity – an essentially relational concept. Because it is dynamic, the challenge for our categorisation and measurement systems is to keep pace with the ever-changing character of opportunity structures and identities. Finally, it is multi-faceted – not least because of the way ethnicity interacts with other principles of identity and stratification. The implication of all of this is that disadvantage is similarly complex. The danger is that we essentialise *ethnic* disadvantage around a restricted concept of ethnicity and fail to capture its interplay with other sources of inclusion and exclusion.

Notes

[1] We should note, however, that apparently novel trends may have deeper roots, as the work of Iganski and Payne (1996, 1999) has suggested.

[2] See the discussions in Donovan (1986); McNaught (1988); Ahmad (1992, 1993); Mason (2000).

THREE

The demographic characteristics of people from minority ethnic groups in Britain

David Owen

Introduction

In recent decades, the existence of a growing population of people from 'minority ethnic groups' within the UK has attracted increasing attention from politicians, policy makers, the media and academia. The minority ethnic groups of policy interest comprise people who are visibly identifiable because their skin colour is brown or black (unlike most European national minorities), and whose family origins lie in the countries of the New Commonwealth: the Indian subcontinent, South East Asia, the Caribbean and Sub-Saharan Africa.

Although small numbers of people with such origins have lived in the UK for centuries, their populations increased dramatically during the second half of the 20th century as a result of high rates of immigration in the 1950s and 1960s, reinforced by high birth rates. Minority ethnic groups now form a significant component of the British population, especially in the younger age groups, and a substantial proportion of the population of London, Birmingham and other major cities. As the pace of globalisation increases and barriers to international travel decline, the diversity of the British population is also increasing as a consequence of new flows of primary migration.

This chapter describes the growth of the minority population, the current ethnic profile of the British population (using data for 1998-2000), the geographical distribution of minority ethnic groups, and the demographic trends underlying the continued growth in the minority population over the medium term[1].

Evolution of the minority ethnic group population

Statistics on the ethnic composition of the British population began to be compiled only from the late 1970s onwards. Therefore, the growth of the minority population from 1945 to 1981 can only be gauged from Census data

on the number of people born outside the UK as well as periodic estimates
made by the Office for Population Censuses and Surveys (OPCS, 1976, 1977).

The initial growth of the minority ethnic group population of Britain began
in the era of mass immigration from the New Commonwealth, which lasted
from the passing of the British Nationality Act in 1948 to the mid-1970s. The
minority ethnic group population of England and Wales increased from 103,000
in 1951 to 415,000 in 1961 (Eversley and Sukdeo, 1969), and to 1.2 million in
1971 (Runnymede Trust and Radical Statistics Race Group, 1980).

The rapid growth of the minority ethnic group population continued,
increasing by around 90,000 per annum during the 1970s and 1980s (Shaw,
1988). Hence, the total population has increased by about a quarter in each
decade. It stood at 2.1 million in 1981 (Labour Force Survey estimates), and
was measured to be 3.1 million by the 1991 Census of Population (the first
census to classify the British population by ethnic group). The 1990s saw
continued growth, and first results from the 2001 Census revealed that the
minority population of the UK was 4.6 million (that is, just over 7% of the
population). Figure 3.1 depicts the steady growth of the minority population
and its growing share of the population of Britain, from 1.7% in 1966-67 to
over 7% at present. The annual rate of growth appears to have accelerated
towards the end of 1990s.

**Figure 3.1: Growth in the minority population of Britain
(1996/97-2000)**

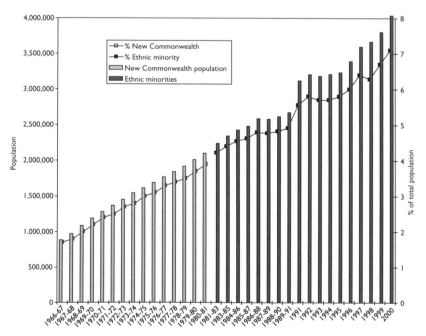

Source: ONS estimates (1966/67-81); Labour Force Survey estimates (1981/83-2000)

Rapid minority population growth has counterbalanced the slow growth (and net emigration for much of the postwar period) of British-born white people. Walker (1977) estimated that immigration increased the total population of England and Wales by 630,000 over the period 1951-76, and that the cumulative number of births due to immigration was 330,000 by 1976. Coleman (1995) estimated that the population of England and Wales in 1991 was around three million greater than it would have been in the absence of the minority ethnic group population. Since then, growth in the white population of Britain has virtually ceased, and the minority population now accounts for almost all the growth in the population of Britain. The components of population change will now be considered in greater detail.

International migration and demographic change

From the end of the Second World War until the early 1980s, with the exception of the peak years of immigration at the beginning and end of the 1960s (which preceded the passing of the Immigration Acts of 1962 and 1968), the number of emigrants leaving the UK exceeded the numbers migrating to the UK. Immigration from the New Commonwealth started in the late 1940s and reached a peak in the late 1950s and early 1960s (Figure 3.2). Immigration

Figure 3.2: Migration from the New Commonwealth to the UK (1955-80)

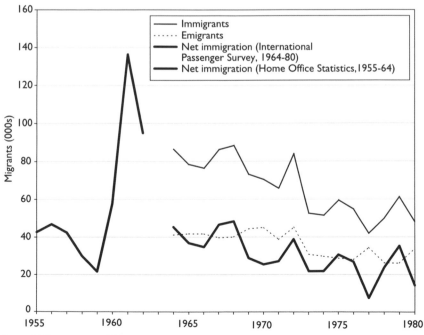

Source: ONS estimates to 1981 then Labour Force Survey

from the Caribbean was largely curtailed by the Commonwealth Immigrants Act of 1962, while the Immigration Act of 1971 had a similar effect upon primary immigration from the Indian subcontinent (Salt, 1996), although the migration of dependants continued. The migration of people from Pakistan and Bangladesh in search of work ended later and the migration of family members from these countries has also lasted longer than the corresponding flows from India and the Caribbean[2].

New flows of migrants developed during the 1980s and 1990s. Initially these flows comprised Chinese (mainly from Hong Kong) and Black–African people (many of whom arrived as students), together with students from other parts of South East Asia. This was followed by the arrival of increasing numbers of asylum seekers (predominantly from Africa, the Middle East, and countries such as Sri Lanka). The revival in net immigration from the New Commonwealth is shown in Figure 3.3, which illustrates both the doubling in the number of immigrants and the decline in the number of emigrants.

Since the early 1980s, the UK has gained population each year through net international migration. The total number of emigrants has remained fairly constant, but the annual number of in-migrants has followed a rising trend. Hence the volume of net immigration has steadily increased. Annual net immigration was around 50,000 throughout most of the 1980s and early 1990s, rose to 100,000 in the late 1980s and 1990s, but exceeded 100,000 in the late 1990s, reaching a peak of 189,000 in 1998-99 (this includes the substantial growth in the number of asylum seekers entering the UK). In total, there was a net gain to the UK population of some 1.2 million people between 1981 and 1999 (Dobson and McLaughlan, 2001, p 30).

Figure 3.3: Migration from the New Commonwealth to the UK (1981-99)

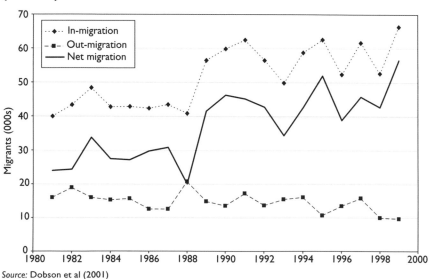

Source: Dobson et al (2001)

There has not only been increased migration from both the 'Old' and 'New' Commonwealths and the rest of the European Union (EU) during the 1990s, but also a substantial increase in migration from the rest of the world. Figure 3.4 demonstrates that the latter has increased faster than other geographical sources of immigration during the past decade, and is now the largest component of net immigration. This increase coincides with the increase in the number of asylum seekers (experienced by all European countries). However, there is clearly an economic influence on this migration flow, since the peaks in migration from the rest of the world (in the late 1980s and late 1990s) coincide with periods of very high UK economic growth. This upward trend in international migration also reflects the falling costs of international travel and increased recruitment of overseas students.

In the most recent set of population projections from the Government Accounting Office (based on data from 2000), the population of the UK is projected to reach 64.7 million by 2025. These projections assume that annual net immigration will be 135,000 for most of this period, accounting for two thirds of total population growth (3.4 million people). With more than two thirds of international migrants settling in Greater London and the South East, these trends imply a substantial increase in pressure on both land for new housing and public service provision in these regions. However, migration trends are very difficult to forecast, and projections of future population are subject to extreme uncertainty as a consequence.

Figure 3.4: Net migration to the UK by citizenship

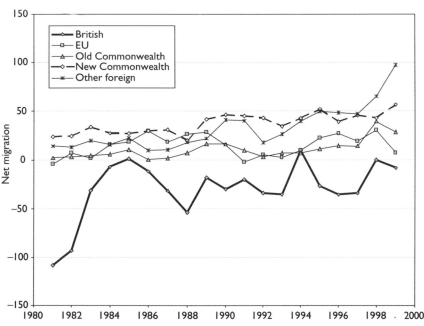

Source: Dobson et al (2001)

Different migrant ethnic groups have entered the UK at different periods in time. Table 3.1 presents percentages of all persons from each ethnic group present in the UK during the period 1998-2000 who entered the country before 1970, between 1970 and 1989, and from 1990 onwards, alongside the percentage of each ethnic group born in the UK. Just over half of all people from minority ethnic groups were born in the UK. Persons of mixed parentage (Black–Mixed and Other–Mixed) are most likely to have been born in the UK, together with the Black–Other ethnic group (mainly people of Caribbean parentage who prefer to describe themselves as 'Black–British'). The percentage of black people born in the UK is greater than that of the South Asian or 'Chinese and Other' ethnic groups, but only just over a third of Black–African people are UK-born.

The concentration of Caribbean migration into the 1960s is revealed by 31.1% of Black–Caribbean people having entered the UK before 1970, while Indian and Pakistani people were more likely to have entered between 1970 and 1989. The peak period of migration for each of these ethnic groups can be clearly seen from Figure 3.5, which plots the date of entry to the UK for people from the main ethnic groupings. Bangladeshi migration is more recent than that of the other South Asian ethnic groups, while two fifths of Black–

Table 3.1: Percentage born in the UK, or entering the UK in each time period (1998-2000)

Labour Force Survey ethnic group	Born in the UK	Pre-1970	Overseas 1970-89	1990 onwards
White	95.5	1.9	1.2	1.4
Minority ethnic groups	**49.5**	**13.2**	**21.3**	**16.0**
Black ethnic groups	58.7	15.3	9.8	16.2
Black–Caribbean	58.5	31.1	5.7	4.7
Black–Mixed	88.6	2.3	3.3	5.8
Black–African	35.3	4.5	20.3	39.9
Black–Other (non-mixed)	89.7	3.4	3.0	3.8
South Asian	47.4	14.6	26.8	11.2
Indian	43.8	18.5	28.5	9.2
Pakistani	53.9	11.6	21.1	13.4
Bangladeshi	44.8	7.6	34.3	13.2
Chinese and Other	40.2	6.9	26.2	26.8
Chinese	26.2	9.6	34.8	29.4
Other–Asian (non-mixed)	19.5	6.4	35.4	38.6
Other–Other (non-mixed)	32.6	4.8	30.7	32.0
Other–Mixed	72.9	7.2	9.3	10.6
All ethnic groups	92.5	2.7	2.5	2.3

Source: Labour Force Survey averages (Spring 1998 to Winter 1999/2000)

Figure 3.5: Number of persons present in 1998-2000 entering the UK in each year by ethnic group

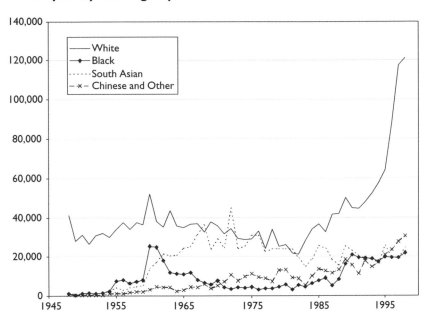

Source: Labour Force Survey (average for Spring 1998 to Winter 1999/2000)

African and Other–Asian (non-mixed) people entered the UK from 1990 onwards. Clearly, international migration is still an important influence on the growth of some minority ethnic groups. Figure 3.5, then, reveals a recent increase in the populations of all three broad minority ethnic groups due to immigration. However, it also reveals that people classified as 'white' have accounted for the greater part of the recent increase in migration[3].

Fertility and mortality

The trend in numbers of births for England and Wales from the Second World War onwards, and in crude birth and death rates (the ratio of births to potential mothers and deaths to the entire population) from 1960 onwards, is depicted in Figure 3.6. The dominant feature of this diagram is the great surge in births in the immediate postwar years and through most of the 1960s. The 1970s was a decade of very low fertility rates, and, following a resurgence of births around 1990s, fertility rates are currently once more in decline. Overall, the number of live births per 1,000 women declined from 91 in 1961 to 57 in 1999 (most of this decline being concentrated among women aged 20-29).

Mortality rates vary very little from year to year, and have described a slow decline throughout this period. As birth rates have declined, the contribution of natural change (births minus deaths) to population increase has therefore

Figure 3.6: Births and deaths in England and Wales (1938-99)

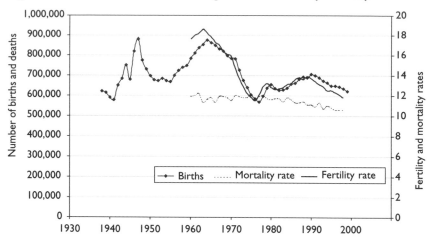

Source: ONS

declined. Natural change was the largest component of population increase during the 1960s, averaging 256,000 per annum between 1957 and 1971. The annual average natural change for the period 1990-99 was 112,000, and had declined to 66,000 by 1999, around a third of the level of net immigration.

Statistics on births and deaths by ethnic group are not collected, but data on the numbers of births by the country of mother's birth are available. These data reveal higher rates of fertility for women born in the New Commonwealth than women born in the UK (and very much higher rates for some ethnic groups). Owen (1995) estimated birth rates and death rates for minority ethnic groups over the period 1981-91 using data from the General Household Survey (Table 3.2). This analysis indicated that minority fertility rates are declining over time, reflecting higher income, occupational mobility and the influence of majority social trends. Fertility decline was greatest for the Caribbean and Indian ethnic groups and least for the Pakistani and Bangladeshi ethnic groups. Fertility rates remain high in those ethnic groups whose migration is recent (for example, Black–African people).

Berthoud (2001) estimated age-specific fertility rates for women from minority ethnic groups using data from the Labour Force Survey for 1987-99. This reveals a complex pattern (Table 3.3): white women are most likely to have children when they reach the 25-29 age group, but women from minority ethnic groups have a more extended period of childbearing. Indian and Pakistani women have higher fertility rates in their early 20s, and Pakistani and Bangladeshi women have children much later in life than white and Indian women. White, Caribbean and Bangladeshi women are most likely to have children as teenagers, but the fertility of older Caribbean women is less than that of women from other ethnic groups. Indian women are most likely to concentrate childbearing into their 20s.

Table 3.2: Britain: change in fertility and mortality rates by ethnic group (1981-91)

Labour Force Survey ethnic group	Mortality rate 1981	1991	Fertility rate 1981	1991
White	12.1	11.7	55.7	57.0
Minority ethnic groups	**2.3**	**2.6**	**90.3**	**84.1**
West Indian	2.1	4.1	35.8	21.2
Indian	2.5	3.6	85.1	70.5
Pakistani	1.2	2.0	204.0	140.5
Bangladeshi	1.3	2.4	254.9	185.5
Chinese	2.9	2.5	79.9	78.9
African	2.2	1.6	126.4	115.6
Arab	1.7	2.9	53.4	74.5
Mixed	2.1	2.0	143.4	160.2
Other	4.6	2.3	25.1	18.8
All ethnic groups	**11.7**	**11.2**	**57.4**	**58.5**

NB: These are crude rates: the mortality rate is deaths per 1,000 population and the fertility rate is births per 1,000 women of childbearing age.

Source: Owen (1995) based on data from the General Household Survey

Mortality rates for many minority ethnic groups are estimated to have increased over the decade. Rates tend to be highest for the ethnic groups with the oldest age structures, notably West Indian and Indian people (Table 3.2). However, there also seems to be a strong association with poverty, since mortality rates for Pakistani and Bangladeshi people also increased, despite the great youth of these ethnic groups. Census data on long-term limiting illness reveals that Chinese people experience the best health of any ethnic group, but that Bangladeshi and Pakistani people have relatively poor health on average. Older Indian people also experience relatively high levels of long-term illness.

Table 3.3: Estimates of fertility by age of mother and ethnic group

Ethnic group	Annual rate per thousand women in the age band					
	15-19	20-24	25-29	30-34	35-39	40-44
White	29	98	125	73	23	5
Caribbean	44	95	104	72	32	9
Indian	17	143	160	95	31	6
Pakistani	41	236	232	160	84	39
Bangladeshi	75	269	272	152	103	74
Other	28	80	129	105	48	11

Source: Berthoud (2001), based on Labour Force Survey data for 1987-99

Table 3.4 presents the geographical distribution of births to mothers born outside the UK. While there is no longer an exact correspondence between country of birth and membership of a minority ethnic group, these figures provide an indication of where births to people from minority ethnic groups and to new immigrants from these groups are located. It also demonstrates the emergence of new minority groups who do not originate from the New Commonwealth. In total, 15% of all births in England and Wales in 2000 were to women born outside the UK, evenly split between mothers born in the New Commonwealth and elsewhere. This indicates that minority ethnic groups will form a growing percentage of the child population across England and Wales, though this high percentage is inflated by the overall decline in the number of births at the end of the 1990s. Nearly half were located in Greater London, of which two fifths of births were to mothers born outside the UK. The majority of all births in Inner London were to mothers born outside the UK. Births to mothers born in the New Commonwealth were a substantial proportion of all births in the West Midlands, West Yorkshire (particularly

Table 3.4: Geographical distribution of births by country of birth of mother (2000)

	All births	New Commonwealth		Rest of the world		All outside United Kingdom	
		Number	%	Number	%	Number	%
North East	26,499	702	3	734	3	1,436	5
North West	76,675	4,423	6	2,757	4	7,180	9
Greater Manchester	*30,401*	*2,750*	*9*	*1,348*	*4*	*4,098*	*13*
Manchester	*5,537*	*691*	*12*	*519*	*9*	*1,210*	*22*
Yorkshire and the Humber	55,966	4,174	7	1,813	3	5,987	11
West Yorkshire	*25,379*	*3,336*	*13*	*712*	*3*	*4,048*	*16*
Bradford	*7,051*	*1,762*	*25*	*176*	*2*	*1,938*	*27*
East Midlands	45,787	2,461	5	1,667	4	4,128	9
West Midlands	61,497	6,033	10	2,043	3	8,076	13
West Midlands	*33,398*	*5,235*	*16*	*1,216*	*4*	*6,451*	*19*
Birmingham	*14,308*	*3,387*	*24*	*637*	*4*	*4,024*	*28*
East	61,186	2,919	5	4,058	7	6,977	11
South East	90,445	4,344	5	6,669	7	11,013	12
Greater London	*104,695*	*20,290*	*19*	*23,134*	*22*	*43,424*	*41*
Inner London	*44,989*	*10,504*	*23*	*12,484*	*28*	*22,988*	*51*
South West	50,076	1,215	2	2,425	5	3,640	7
Wales	31,304	651	2	951	3	1,602	5
England and Wales	**604,130**	**47,212**	**8**	**46,251**	**8**	**93,463**	**15**

Source: Labour Force Survey (average for Spring 1998 to Winter 1999/2000)

Bradford) and Greater Manchester. Births to mothers born elsewhere in the world were more concentrated within Greater London. This geographical pattern indicates continued substantial growth of the minority population in these major cities, but also suggests that these minority ethnic groups remain geographically concentrated.

Structure of the minority population

At the end of the 20th century, the minority ethnic group population of the UK was approaching four million, representing 6.6% of the total population of 58.5 million. While the Caribbean population was initially the largest and fastest-growing minority ethnic group, migrants from the Indian subcontinent soon followed, and the Indian population had overtaken the Caribbean population to become the largest individual ethnic group by 1981[4]. In 1991 the relative position of these two ethnic groups was maintained, but the Pakistani ethnic group had grown to become the third largest. The average ethnic composition of the UK over the period 1998-2000 is presented in Table 3.5. The South Asian ethnic groups comprise over 1.8 million people (3.2% of the

Table 3.5: Ethnic composition of the UK (average for 1998-2000)

	Male	Female	Persons	%	Males per 1,000 females
White	26,948,956	27,754,234	54,703,190	93.4	971
Minority ethnic groups	**1,931,299**	**1,916,446**	**3,847,744**	**6.6**	**1,008**
Black	585,629	618,280	1,203,909	2.1	947
Black–Caribbean	241,192	266,994	508,186	0.9	903
Black–Mixed	92,700	91,755	184,455	0.3	1,010
Black–Other (non-mixed)	58,329	61,644	119,972	0.2	946
Black–African	193,408	197,887	391,296	0.7	977
South Asian	953,677	891,128	1,844,805	3.2	1,070
Indian	487,431	468,326	955,757	1.6	1,041
Pakistani	328,848	306,616	635,464	1.1	1,073
Bangladeshi	137,399	116,185	253,584	0.4	1,183
Chinese and Other	391,993	407,038	799,030	1.4	963
Chinese	72,479	79,601	152,080	0.3	911
Other–Asian (non-mixed)	101,734	114,372	216,106	0.4	890
Other–Other (non-mixed)	99,597	87,226	186,823	0.3	1,142
Other–Mixed	118,183	125,839	244,021	0.4	939
All ethnic groups	**28,880,254**	**29,670,679**	**58,550,934**	**100.0**	**973**

Source: Labour Force Survey (average for Spring 1998 to Winter 1999/2000)

total). Black ethnic groups comprise 2.1% of the total population of the UK, with the Black–Caribbean ethnic group now the third largest ethnic group. The Black–African ethnic group has overtaken the Bangladeshi ethnic group in size, while the Chinese is the smallest of the main ethnic groups. People of mixed parentage now form 0.7% of the population. Males are just in the majority among people from minority ethnic groups as a whole, with the greatest excess of males over females occurring in the Bangladeshi, Other – Other (non-mixed) and Pakistani ethnic groups. In contrast, females form the majority of Black–Caribbean people. The female share of each ethnic group has increased since 1991.

Table 3.6 presents estimates of population change by ethnic group between 1991 and 1999 (these do not quite match the actual data for 1998-2000 and underestimate international migration). These are created by ageing forward the 1991 population of each ethnic and age group, based on the known pattern of overall population change. The minority population is estimated to have increased by about two thirds of a million during the 1990s (21.3%), while the white population remained more or less constant. Rates of increase were greatest in the smaller, more recent and mixed parentage ethnic groups, and the Black–Other and Black–African ethnic groups both grew by two thirds. The increase in the total population was greatest for the Pakistani ethnic group, but this only narrowly exceeded the growth of the Black–African ethnic group. The demography of the Indian ethnic group indicated that its rate of increase

Table 3.6: Estimated population change (1991-99)

Ethnic group	1991 population (000s)	1999 population (000s)	Change (000s)	% change
White	53,084.7	53,074.2	-10.5	0.0
Minority ethnic groups	**3,121.9**	**3,787.2**	**665.4**	**21.3**
Black	*9,26.0*	*1,174.7*	*2,48.8*	*26.9*
Caribbean	703.6	798.5	94.9	13.5
Black–Caribbean	517.7	490.1	-27.6	-5.3
Black–Other	185.9	308.4	122.5	65.9
Black–African	222.4	376.2	153.9	69.2
South Asian	*1,528.0*	*1,860.4*	*332.5*	*21.8*
Indian	866.3	929.6	63.3	7.3
Pakistani	493.2	662.9	169.7	34.4
Bangladeshi	168.5	267.9	99.5	59.0
Chinese and Other	*667.9*	*752.0*	*84.1*	*12.6*
Chinese	162.8	136.7	−26.0	−16.0
Other–Asian	204.2	206.4	2.2	1.1
Other–Other	300.9	408.9	108.0	35.9
All ethnic groups	**56,206.5**	**56,879.4**	**672.9**	**1.2**

Source: Owen et al (2000)

Table 3.7:Age structure of each ethnic group (1998-2000)

Ethnic group	0-15	16-17	18-24	25-34	35-49	50-59	60+
				Age group			
White	19.8	2.4	8.2	15.0	21.3	12.5	20.7
Minority ethnic groups	*31.5*	*3.4*	*11.7*	*17.5*	*21.6*	*6.5*	*7.8*
Black	*33.8*	*3.2*	*10.2*	*17.8*	*21.3*	*5.6*	*8.0*
Black–Caribbean	22.8	2.6	8.8	16.7	25.0	8.7	15.4
Black–Mixed	61.1	4.2	11.3	11.8	8.9	1.4	1.3
Black–Other (non-mixed)	43.4	4.3	11.5	20.1	17.6	1.1	2.1
Black–African	32.4	3.2	11.3	21.4	23.5	4.7	3.5
South Asian	*30.0*	*3.7*	*12.5*	*17.0*	*21.1*	*6.7*	*8.8*
Indian	23.5	3.1	11.1	17.1	25.3	8.9	10.9
Pakistani	35.6	4.3	13.9	17.5	17.5	4.6	6.6
Bangladeshi	40.6	4.7	14.3	15.3	14.4	4.2	6.6
Chinese and Other	*31.4*	*3.0*	*12.2*	*17.9*	*23.0*	*7.6*	*5.0*
Chinese	16.8	2.9	16.9	19.6	26.6	8.9	8.2
Other–Asian (non-mixed)	19.5	2.1	10.8	21.9	30.7	9.6	5.5
Other–Other (non-mixed)	27.3	3.2	12.3	18.4	26.2	8.6	4.1
Other–Mixed	54.1	3.6	10.3	13.1	11.4	4.1	3.4
All ethnic groups	**20.6**	**2.5**	**8.4**	**15.2**	**21.3**	**12.1**	**19.9**

Source: Labour Force Survey (average for Spring 1998 to Winter 1999/2000)

would slow markedly during the decade, while the population of the Black–Caribbean and Chinese ethnic groups were set to stabilise or decline.

Table 3.7 presents the age breakdown of each ethnic group during the period 1998-2000. Minority ethnic groups are more youthful on average than white people, with nearly a third of the minority population of less than compulsory school-leaving age. Conversely, one fifth of the white population is of pensionable age, compared with one in 12 of the minority population. The Black Caribbean population is the most elderly minority ethnic group, with 15.4% of its population of pensionable age. Both these ethnic groups will contain substantial numbers of elderly people from the second decade of the 21st century onwards. The Pakistani population is maturing, with only a third now aged 0-15. The most youthful ethnic groups are the Black–Mixed and Other–Other (mixed) ethnic groups, more than half of which are aged under 16.

The minority share of each age group declines with increasing age (Table 3.8). One tenth of children and just over 9% of those of an age to enter the labour market are from minority ethnic groups, but only 2.6% of those aged 60+ are from minority ethnic groups. The Black–Caribbean share of each age group remains constant at around 1% of the population until the age of 50, while the decline in population share occurs earlier in the age range for South Asian ethnic groups, demonstrating their greater relative youth. The population share for ethnic groups of mixed parentage declines most rapidly with increasing age.

Table 3.8: Ethnic composition of each age group (1998-2000)

	% of the total UK population of each age group						
Ethnic group	0-15	16-17	18-24	25-34	35-49	50-59	60+
White	90.0	90.9	90.8	92.4	93.3	96.5	97.4
Minority ethnic groups	**10.0**	**9.1**	**9.2**	**7.6**	**6.7**	**3.5**	**2.6**
Black	*3.4*	*2.7*	*2.5*	*2.4*	*2.1*	*0.9*	*0.8*
Black–Caribbean	1.0	0.9	0.9	1.0	1.0	0.6	0.7
Black–Mixed	0.9	0.5	0.4	0.2	0.1	0.0	0.0
Black–Other (non-mixed)	0.4	0.4	0.3	0.3	0.2	0.0	0.0
Black–African	1.1	0.9	0.9	0.9	0.7	0.3	0.1
South Asian	*4.6*	*4.8*	*4.7*	*3.5*	*3.1*	*1.7*	*1.4*
Indian	1.9	2.1	2.2	1.8	1.9	1.2	0.9
Pakistani	1.9	1.9	1.8	1.3	0.9	0.4	0.4
Bangladeshi	0.9	0.8	0.7	0.4	0.3	0.2	0.1
Chinese and Other	*2.1*	*1.6*	*2.0*	*1.6*	*1.5*	*0.8*	*0.3*
Chinese	0.2	0.3	0.5	0.3	0.3	0.2	0.1
Other–Asian (non-mixed)	0.3	0.3	0.5	0.5	0.5	0.3	0.1
Other–Other (non-mixed)	0.4	0.4	0.5	0.4	0.4	0.2	0.1
Other–Mixed	1.1	0.6	0.5	0.4	0.2	0.1	0.1
All ethnic groups	**100.0**	**100.0**	**100.0**	**100.0**	**100.0**	**100.0**	**100.0**

Source: Labour Force Survey (average for Spring 1998 to Winter 1999/2000)

Household and family structure

Household size is similar for people from the white and Caribbean ethnic groups, but Black–African, Chinese and Indian households are rather larger, and Pakistani and Bangladeshi households are on average twice the size of white households (Table 3.9). There are major differences in family organisation between ethnic groups. The percentage of people living alone is highest for white and Caribbean people, but in the former case this is influenced by the higher percentage of pensioners. Cohabiting and other non-traditional forms of partnership are most common for the white and Caribbean ethnic groups. Single-parent families are more common in the Black–Caribbean ethnic group than for other minority ethnic groups (accounting for more than two fifths of all families, compared with only one tenth of South Asian families and 13.1% of white families), and marriage is also less common and later in this ethnic group. Family patterns among young Caribbean people are more similar to those in the West Indies than in the migrant generation. Marriage is most common in the South Asian ethnic groups, and age of marriage is also relatively low in these ethnic groups.

Nearly a quarter of all black households consisted of single non-pensioner adults, and this household type was more than twice as common for these ethnic groups than for white households. They were also common in the

Table 3.9: Household and family composition for black and white ethnic groups in Britain (1991)

Household characteristics or family type	White	Minority ethnic groups	Black	Black–Caribbean	Black–African	Black–Other	All South Asian	Indian	Paki-stani	Bagla-deshi	Chinese and Other	Chin-ese	Other–Asian	Other–Other
All households (100%)	21,026,565	870,757	328,087	216,460	73,346	38,281	357,188	225,582	100,938	30,668	185,482	48,619	58,955	77,908
Mean household size	2.4	3.3	2.6	2.5	2.8	2.5	4.2	3.8	4.8	5.3	3.0	3.1	3.2	2.7
Mean number of dependent children	1.8	2.2	1.8	1.8	2.0	1.8	2.5	2.1	3.0	3.4	2.0	2.0	1.9	2.0
Percent pensioner households	25.7	4.2	5.6	7.2	2.0	1.8	2.8	3.6	1.4	1.0	4.4	3.7	2.6	6.2
All families (10% sample)	1,462,155	83,095	20,930	14,098	4,289	2,543	34,064	21,364	9,758	2,942	13,002	3,462	4,456	5,084
Married couple families	79.2	74.2	48.3	47.3	55.0	42.9	88.5	89.6	86.8	86.4	78.4	84.8	82.7	70.2
With no dependent children	35.6	17.1	14.1	15.6	13.5	11.9	17.5	20.6	13.4	8.2	20.2	21.8	19.3	19.9
With one or more dependent children	25.0	49.0	31.1	20.3	39.1	27.0	62.9	58.8	68.0	75.1	51.4	55.8	56.8	43.7
With non-dependent children	12.5	8.1	8.6	11.4	2.3	4.0	8.2	10.1	5.5	3.0	6.8	7.3	6.6	6.6

Table 3.9: contd.../

Household characteristics or family type	White	Minority ethnic groups	Black	Black-Caribbean	Black-African	Black-Other	All South Asian	Indian	Pakistani	Bangladeshi	Chinese and Other	Chinese	Other-Asian	Other-Other
Cohabiting couple families	7.7	4.9	10.3	10.7	7.2	13.7	1.3	1.4	1.1	0.8	5.4	3.4	3.4	8.6
With no dependent children	4.9	2.6	5.1	5	4	7.3	0.7	0.9	0.6	0.4	3.6	2.5	2.2	5.6
With one or more dependent children	2.5	2.1	4.9	5.2	3.1	6.3	0.5	0.5	0.5	0.4	1.7	0.8	1.1	2.8
With non-dependent children	0.3	0.2	0.4	0.6	0.1	0.1	0	0	0.1	0	0.1	0.1	0.1	0.2
Lone-parent families	13.1	20.9	41.3	42	37.9	43.4	10.2	9	12	12.8	16.2	11.8	13.8	21.2
With one or more dependent children	32.3	15.8	7.8	30.8	33.5	38.9	7	5.4	9.4	11.3	12.2	8.1	10	17
With non-dependent children	5.4	5.1	9	11.2	4.4	4.5	3.2	3.6	2.6	1.5	3.9	3.7	3.8	4.2

Source: 1991 Census of Population (ESRC/JISC purchase)

Other–Other (22%) and Chinese (18.8%) ethnic groups. In contrast, 25.7% of white households contained pensioners, compared with only 4.2% of all households from minority ethnic groups.

In 1991, couples without children (where there had either never been any children or where children had left the family home) were more than twice as common (29.5%) among white-headed households than minority ethnic group households (13.3%), being least common among Pakistani and Bangladeshi households. Large families without children (three or more adults and no dependent children) were most prevalent in Indian (13.4%), Black–Caribbean (11.4%) and white (11.1%) households representing either families with older children who had not yet left home, or the presence of older relatives living with a couple. Small families (couples with dependent children) were most common for Bangladeshi (43.3%), Pakistani (41%), Indian (36.4%) and Other Asian (34.7%) households, and least common for Black Caribbean households (14.8%).

Geography

Migrants from the New Commonwealth who came to Britain in the 1950s and 1960s in search of work tended to settle in London, Birmingham and other industrial cities and towns of the Midlands and the North of England, where jobs in manufacturing industry and public sector services were readily available. In spite of the general tendency for people to leave the cities and move to smaller towns and rural areas, and the massive loss of jobs in the larger urban areas, people from minority ethnic groups have remained geographically concentrated into the major cities (Owen, 1997). Table 3.10 demonstrates that the share of minority ethic groups in the main areas of settlement steadily increased over the period 1971-91, at the same time as these regions and metropolitan counties were losing population in relative terms to the areas of more recent employment growth (notably East Anglia and South West England).

The Labour Force Survey for the period 1998-2000 is used in Table 3.11 to describe the current regional distribution of people from minority ethnic groups. Of the minority ethnic group population of 3.9 million, almost half (48.3%) live in Greater London and an eighth in the West Midlands (former) metropolitan county. Outside these two major conurbations, the largest minority populations are located in the Greater Manchester and West Yorkshire (former) metropolitan counties. In comparison, only one tenth of all white people live in Greater London and 3.9% live in the West Midlands, graphically illustrating the degree of spatial segregation between people from white and minority ethnic groups.

Nearly two thirds of people from the three black ethnic groups live in Greater London, with a further eighth living in the West Midlands. In contrast, only just over one third of South Asian people lived in the Greater London area in the period 1998-2000 (and were more likely to live in Greater London as a whole than Inner London). The West Midlands was a more important

Table 3.10: Minority population change by region (1971-91)

Region, country or metropolitan county (MC)	Total population		Minority ethnic group population			
	Population 1991	% change 1971-91	1971 (%)	1981 (%)	1991 (%)	(000s)
South East	17,208.3	5.5	4.3	7.4	9.9	1,695.4
Greater London	6,679.7	-7.4	7.9	14.3	20.2	1,346.1
East Anglia	2,027.0	26.1	0.7	1.5	2.1	43.4
South West	4,609.4	18.2	0.8	1.5	1.3	62.6
West Midlands	5,150.2	3.0	4.1	6.4	8.2	424.4
West Midlands MC	2,551.7	-7.1	6.8	10.9	14.6	373.5
East Midlands	3,953.4	11.4	2.0	3.7	4.8	188.0
Yorkshire and Humberside	4,836.5	1.4	1.9	3.2	4.5	214.0
West Yorkshire	2,013.7	-0.5	3.4	5.9	8.2	164.1
North West	6,243.7	-3.1	1.3	2.7	3.9	244.6
Greater Manchester	2,499.4	-6.9	2.1	3.9	5.9	148.2
North	3,026.7	-1.4	0.4	0.9	1.3	38.5
Tyne and Wear	1,095.2	-8.0	0.4	1.0	1.8	19.9
Wales	2,835.1	6.6	0.4	0.9	1.5	41.6
Scotland	4,998.6	-1.1	0.4	*	1.2	62.6
Great Britain	54,888.8	4.8	2.4	4.2	5.5	3,015.1

Note: * The 1981 Scottish Census did not collect these data.

Source: 1971, 1981 and 1991 Censuses of Population (Owen, 1993)

concentration for South Asians than other ethnic groups. However, Schuman (1999) demonstrated that there were major differences in the geographical distribution of the three South Asian ethnic groups in 1997. Around half of all Bangladeshis lived in Greater London, but Pakistani people were much more likely to live in northern England and the Midlands. Indian people had a more geographically widespread distribution than people from the other two South Asian ethnic groups. Chinese people were less strongly concentrated geographically than people from other minority ethnic groups.

The ethnic composition of Greater London is very different from that of the rest of Britain. A quarter of its overall population and one third of Inner London's population are from minority ethnic groups. Only the West Midlands (former) metropolitan county approached this percentage, with over a sixth of its population being from minority ethnic groups. Black people formed the largest part of the minority population of Greater London, while South Asian people comprised the largest minority groups in the West Midlands. Elsewhere, only in Greater Manchester did the minority share of the population exceed the UK average. In Wales, Scotland and the peripheral regions of England, minority ethnic groups still formed less than 2% of the resident population.

Unfortunately, the Labour Force Survey is based upon too small a sample to yield reliable information on the detailed geographical distribution of minority ethnic groups. Therefore, at the time of writing, the 1991 Census of Population

Table 3.11: Percentage share of resident population from minority ethnic groups (1998-2000)

Region/country/ metropolitan county (MC)	Total population	Minority ethnic groups	% of resident population			Regional share of UK population				
			Black	South Asian	Chinese and Other	White	Minority	Black	South Asian	Chinese and Other
North East	2,551,693	1.7	0.2	1.0	0.5	4.6	1.1	0.5	1.4	1.5
Tyne and Wear MC	1,100,072	2.4	–	1.5	0.6	2.0	0.7	–	0.9	0.9
North West	6,787,583	4.1	0.8	2.6	0.7	11.9	7.2	4.4	9.6	5.7
Greater Manchester MC	2,546,791	6.9	1.4	4.4	1.0	4.3	4.6	3.0	6.1	3.3
Yorkshire and Humberside	4,983,266	5.6	1.0	3.8	0.8	8.6	7.2	4.3	10.2	4.9
West Yorkshire MC	2,092,070	10.2	1.6	7.6	1.1	3.4	5.6	2.7	8.6	2.8
East Midlands	4,137,762	4.7	1.1	3.0	0.6	7.2	5.1	3.8	6.8	3.0
West Midlands	5,275,902	9.9	2.2	6.8	0.9	8.7	13.6	9.7	19.5	5.7
West Midlands MC	2,596,768	17.9	3.8	12.7	1.4	3.9	12.1	8.2	17.9	4.4
Eastern	5,339,888	3.7	1.0	1.9	0.9	9.4	5.2	4.3	5.4	5.8
Greater London	7,121,126	26.1	10.8	9.4	5.9	9.6	48.3	63.8	36.3	52.7
Inner London	2,721,959	31.8	16.8	8.0	7.0	3.4	22.5	38.1	11.8	23.7
Outer London	4,399,167	22.6	7.0	10.3	5.3	6.2	25.8	25.7	24.5	29.0
Rest of South East	7,914,743	3.4	0.8	1.5	1.1	14.0	6.9	5.0	6.3	11.3
South West	4,832,118	1.5	0.5	0.5	0.5	8.7	1.9	2.1	1.3	3.2
Wales	2,899,233	1.7	0.5	0.5	0.7	5.2	1.3	1.1	0.7	2.7
Scotland	5,039,964	1.6	0.2	0.8	0.5	9.1	2.0	0.8	2.3	3.2
Strathclyde	2,236,554	2.2	0.2	1.4	0.6	4.0	1.3	0.4	1.8	1.6
Northern Ireland	1,667,656	0.3	–	–	–	3.0	0.1	–	–	–
UK	58,550,934	6.6	2.1	3.2	1.4	100.0	100.0	100.0	100.0	100.0

Note: Counts of less than 3,000 have been suppressed.

Source: Labour Force Survey (average for Spring 1998 to Winter 1999/2000)

is still the best source of such data. This revealed that the London boroughs (notably Brent, Newham and Tower Hamlets) contained some of the largest local concentrations of minority ethnic groups. Table 3.12 presents the 20 local authority districts collectively containing 55.2% of all people from minority ethnic groups in 1991. Outside London, the major concentrations of minority ethnic groups occurred in Leicester, Slough, Birmingham, Luton, Wolverhampton, Bradford and Blackburn (Owen, 1992; Rees and Phillips, 1996).

Table 3.12: Largest local concentrations of people from minority ethnic groups (1991)

Local authority district	Minority ethnic groups				
	% of locality	Population (000s)	% of Britain	Largest minority group	% share of population
Brent	44.8	108.9	3.6	Indian	17.2
Newham	42.3	89.8	3.0	Indian	13.0
Tower Hamlets	35.6	57.3	1.9	Bangladeshi	22.9
Hackney	33.6	60.8	2.0	Black–Caribbean	11.2
Ealing	32.3	88.9	3.0	Indian	16.1
Lambeth	30.3	74.1	2.5	Black–Caribbean	12.6
Haringey	29.0	58.7	2.0	Black–Caribbean	9.3
Leicester	28.5	77.0	2.6	Indian	22.3
Slough	27.7	28.0	0.9	Indian	12.5
Harrow	26.2	52.4	1.7	Indian	16.1
Waltham Forest	25.6	54.2	1.8	Black–Caribbean	6.8
Southwark	24.4	53.4	1.8	Black–Caribbean	8.3
Hounslow	24.4	49.9	1.7	Indian	14.3
Lewisham	22.0	50.7	1.7	Black–Caribbean	10.1
Birmingham	21.5	206.8	6.9	Pakistani	6.9
Westminster, City of	21.4	37.4	1.2	Other–Other	4.3
Redbridge	21.4	48.4	1.6	Indian	10.2
Wandsworth	20.0	50.6	1.7	Black–Caribbean	6.1
Luton	19.8	34.0	1.1	Pakistani	6.2
Islington	18.9	31.1	1.0	Black–Caribbean	5.1
Wolverhampton	18.6	45.0	1.5	Indian	11.4
Barnet	18.4	54.0	1.8	Indian	7.3
Camden	17.8	30.4	1.0	Bangladeshi	3.5
Croydon	17.6	55.1	1.9	Black–Caribbean	4.9
Hammersmith and Fulham	17.5	26.0	0.9	Black–Caribbean	5.9
Merton	16.3	27.4	0.9	Indian	3.4
Bradford	15.6	71.3	2.4	Pakistani	9.9
Kensington and Chelsea	15.6	21.6	0.7	Other–Other	3.6
Blackburn	15.4	21.0	0.7	Indian	7.7
Total		**1,664.2**	**55.2**		

Source: 1991 Census of Population (ESRC/JISC purchase)

Owen (1999) estimated the geographical pattern of population change between 1991 and 1996 for local authority districts in England and Wales by ageing the 1991 population classified by ethnic group, age and gender forward in line with overall population trends. The largest estimated population increases are presented in Table 3.13.

The largest estimated increases in the white population occurred in areas of rapid economic growth, such as Oxford, Cambridge and Milton Keynes. Cities such as Birmingham, Bradford, Leicester and Manchester, together with London boroughs, dominated minority population change. Birmingham's minority population is estimated to have increased by over 23,000, mainly as a result of the 15,000 increase in the number of South Asian people. The growth of black ethnic groups was greatest in London boroughs. For South Asians, the largest estimated population increases outside Birmingham occurred in West Yorkshire. For the 'Chinese and Other' ethnic groups, population increases were estimated to be greatest in Birmingham, Leeds, Manchester and Inner London boroughs.

Geographical segregation

Spatial statistics have been used to summarise the tendency of minority ethnic groups to be concentrated in particular areas and the degree to which they have contact with the majority ethnic group, represented by spatial proximity. The most commonly used measure in the literature concerning the spatial segregation of black and white people is the *Index of Dissimilarity*, which measures the percentage of the 'black' population who would have to move their residence for the spatial distribution to match that of white people (Peach, 1975, 1996).

An alternative is Lieberson's index (Lieberson, 1980) which measures the probability of a member of a given ethnic group coming into contact with a member of another group. The larger that group's share of the overall population of a city, the greater the probability of contact between a minority ethnic group and another ethnic group (or with itself). This is taken account of by subtracting the proportion of the city's population represented by an ethnic group from the value of the index. A positive value on this measure for a minority ethnic group relative to white people would indicate that the minority ethnic group is relatively dispersed among the white population, while a negative value indicates geographical concentration of the minority. The greater the negative value, the greater the degree of concentration into areas where the percentage of the population from the minority ethnic group is relatively high.

These two indices were calculated for 1981 and 1991 using estimates for 1981 and Census data for 1991 for all 9,527 electoral wards in England and Wales. In 1981, the Index of Dissimilarity revealed a high degree of spatial separation. Nearly 80% of Bangladeshi and Pakistani people, three quarters of Black–Caribbean and Black–African people, and two thirds of Indian people would have had to move for their geographical distribution to be the same as that of white people. The Chinese were less segregated than any other minority ethnic group, but even for this ethnic group, almost half its members would

Table 3.13: Largest estimated population increases by ethnic group (1991-96)

White		Minority ethnic groups (000s)		Black (000s)		South Asian (000s)		Chinese and Other (000s)	
Oxford	19.0	Birmingham	23.3	Lambeth	5.9	Birmingham	15.2	Birmingham	3.4
Cambridge	18.6	Tower Hamlets	9.6	Birmingham	4.8	Bradford	7.9	Westminster, City of	2.9
Cardiff	17.0	Ealing	9.5	Southwark	4.0	Tower Hamlets	7.8	Barnet	2.7
Milton Keynes	16.3	Bradford	9.4	Hackney	3.3	Leicester	7.2	Ealing	2.0
Richmond-upon-Thames	14.2	Newham	9.2	Haringey	2.8	Ealing	5.4	Kensington and Chelsea	1.6
Leeds	13.8	Leicester	9.2	Newham	2.8	Newham	5.4	Leeds	1.4
Westminster, City of	12.9	Lambeth	7.7	Lewisham	2.8	Kirklees	4.0	Manchester	1.4
Barnet	11.9	Westminster, City of	7.3	Westminster, City of	2.7	Slough	3.2	Camden	1.3
Bracknell Forest	11.8	Barnet	6.9	Croydon	2.7	Harrow	3.2	Croydon	1.3
Kensington and Chelsea	10.9	Manchester	5.6	Ealing	2.2	Leeds	2.9	Lambeth	1.2

Table 3.14: England and Wales: change in segregation of minority ethnic groups compared with white people (1981-91)

Ethnic group	Index of Dissimilarity			Excess probability of contact with white people		
	1981	1991	Change	1981	1991	Change
Minority ethnic groups	**61.9**	**61.6**	**–0.3**	**–0.175**	**–0.203**	**0.028**
Black	69.1	67.7	–1.4	–0.174	–0.195	0.021
Black–Caribbean	72.4	71.4	–1.0	–0.186	–0.210	0.024
Black–African	73.7	73.8	0.1	–0.166	–0.204	0.038
Black–Other	60.9	57.6	–3.3	–0.138	–0.142	0.004
South Asian	68.0	68.1	0.1	–0.211	–0.246	0.035
Indian	67.2	67.2	0.0	–0.211	–0.238	0.027
Pakistani	77.7	77.2	–0.5	–0.216	–0.257	0.041
Bangladeshi	79.5	76.5	–3.0	–0.197	–0.257	0.060
Chinese and Other	48.8	48.3	–0.5	–0.092	–0.112	0.020
Chinese	47.2	45.0	–2.2	–0.062	–0.073	0.011
Other–Asian	60.2	60.6	0.4	–0.120	–0.150	0.030
Other–Other	47.6	46.9	–0.7	–0.090	–0.106	0.016

have had to move for its geographical distribution to match that of white people. Two ethnic groups with a relatively large percentage of British-born people and people of mixed parentage – Black–Other and Other–Other – displayed relatively low values for the Index of Dissimilarity.

There was little change over the period 1981-91, since the percentage of people from minority ethnic groups who would have to move for their geographical distribution to be the same as that of white people declined by only 0.3%. Within this overall average, African-Caribbean ethnic groups had a slightly more similar geographical distribution to white people in 1991 than in 1981. The largest reduction in segregation was for the Black–Other ethnic group, for which the percentage of the population, which would have to move for its geographical distribution to be the same as white people, fell by 3.3%. The degree of change in segregation was smaller for South Asian people as a whole, but the segregation level of the Bangladeshi ethnic group fell by 3%. Among other minority ethnic groups, the reduction in the degree of segregation was greatest for Chinese people (2%); on the other hand, the degree of segregation increased marginally for the Black–African and Other–Asian ethnic groups.

However, Lieberson's Index indicates that the degree of geographical concentration of individual minority ethnic groups was increasing slightly during the decade. The probability of contact between people from minority ethnic groups as a whole and white people was –0.175 in 1981. This indicates that the chance of a person from a minority ethnic group having a white neighbour was 17.5% less than would be the case were people from minority ethnic groups distributed across England and Wales in the same way as white people. This value fell by 0.028 between 1981 and 1991, which means that the probability of a person from a minority ethnic group having a white neighbour was 2.8% less in 1991 than it was in 1981 (more than 20% smaller than would be the case were white people and minority ethnic groups located in the same areas). In 1991, the three South Asian ethnic groups were the most isolated of all minority ethnic groups from white people, with the probability of contact with white people being about 25% less than if their spatial distribution had been the same as for white people. The probability of having a white neighbour was greatest for the Chinese ethnic group.

The decline in this probability between 1981 and 1991 was greatest for the Pakistani, Bangladeshi and Black–African ethnic groups, three of the fastest growing ethnic groups. The probability of contact between Bangladeshi and white people was 6% less in 1991 than in 1981, with the reduction in this probability being 4.1% for Pakistani people and 3.8% for Black–African people. All minority ethnic groups experienced a reduction in the probability of having a white neighbour over the period 1981-91, but this reduction was smallest for the Black–Other, Chinese and Other–Other ethnic groups.

The list of districts with the highest Indices of Dissimilarity (Table 3.15) is dominated by smaller towns and places remote from the main concentrations of minority ethnic groups. Many of these are extremely rural areas, such as Craven or Berwick-upon-Tweed, with very small minority populations. This list also contains areas with military bases, such as Suffolk Coastal (which would have contained most of its minority residents). However, the Pennine mill towns such as Burnley, Rochdale, Oldham and Bradford, with significant minority populations, are also prominent. Indices of Dissimilarity for black people were highest in the rural areas, with small populations probably concentrated within the urban parts of these fairly sparsely populated districts. The largest city to appear in this list is Leeds, with an Index of Dissimilarity of 61.2. For South Asians, the highest Indices of Dissimilarity occurred in more remote districts, but not all of these were rural (for example, Barrow-in-Furness). For Indian people, Indices of Dissimilarity were much higher in less populous rural areas than in smaller manufacturing towns. However, the ranking of index values identifies two notable concentrations of Indian people – Ealing and Blackburn, both districts in which Indians dominate certain residential areas (such as Southall in Ealing). For Pakistani people, the Index of Dissimilarity identifies a pattern of local concentrations of this ethnic group in smaller manufacturing and industrial towns (such as Langbaurgh, Rhymney Valley, Derby, Peterborough). Districts in South Wales and North East England are quite common in this list. Indices of Dissimilarity for 'Chinese and Other' people were highest in the most rural areas.

In 1991, the pattern of dissimilarity at the district scale was dominated by larger towns and cities, particularly those located around the Pennines (Table 3.16). At least half of the minority population in districts with the 15 largest

Table 3.15: Local authority districts with largest Indices of Dissimilarity by ethnic group (1981)

All minorities		Black		South Asian		Indian		Pakistani		Chinese and Other	
Craven	73.3	73.3	King's Lynn and West Norfolk	81.9	Craven	93.3	Rutland	77.6	Craven	70.6	Berwick-upon-Tweed
East Staffordshire	65.4	65.4	Hyndburn	76.4	Rutland	77.6	Copeland	77.0	Langbaurgh-on-Tees	62.6	South Northamptonshire
England and Wales	61.9	61.9	Arfon	74.3	Copeland	77.0	Barrow-in-Furness	76.4	Halton	60.5	South Hams
Burnley	61.9	61.9	Selby	73.9	Barrow-in-Furness	76.4	Ceredigion	70.2	Rhymney Valley	60.1	Allerdale
Rotherham	61.7	61.7	Suffolk Coastal	72.5	Rotherham	72.9	Arfon	70.0	Derby	58.0	Ceredigion
Bolton	61.2	61.2	Mid-Bedfordshire	70.4	East Staffordshire	71.8	Preseli Pembrokeshire	68.4	East Staffordshire	57.3	Teesdale
Suffolk Coastal	61.1	61.1	Derwentside	70.1	Oldham	68.9	Caradon	67.7	Rotherham	55.4	Cherwell
Rochdale	60.8	60.8	England and Wales	69.1	England and Wales	68.0	England and Wales	67.2	England and Wales	54.8	Mid-Bedfordshire
Blackburn	60.5	60.5	Trafford	67.6	Caradon	67.7	South Derbyshire	66.8	Huntingdonshire	54.8	Forest Heath
Forest Heath	60.4	60.4	Carlisle	66.9	Rochdale	67.6	Bolton	66.7	Chiltern	53.9	South Shropshire
Oldham	60.0	60.0	Holderness	65.7	Ceredigion	67.2	South Lakeland	65.7	Oldham	53.7	Hart
Pendle	58.6	58.6	Cherwell	64.6	South Derbyshire	66.8	Wychavon	65.2	Peterborough	52.3	North Shropshire
Berwick-upon-Tweed	58.3	58.3	Restormel	63.1	Derby	66.6	South Holland	62.9	Blaenau Gwent	52.1	Castle Morpeth
Calderdale	57.9	57.9	Forest Heath	62.9	Bolton	65.9	Ealing	62.9	Stockton-on-Tees	50.5	Preseli Pembrokeshire
Bradford	57.6	57.6	South Northamptonshire	61.5	South Lakeland	65.7	Blackburn	62.3	Port Talbot	49.8	Brecknock
Derby	57.4	57.4	Leeds	61.2	Calderdale	65.7	Carmarthen	61.8	Southampton	49.2	Oswestry

index values would have to move were their distribution to match that of white people. Black people again experienced high levels of segregation in rural areas with military bases (Suffolk Coastal and Richmondshire) or large educational establishments (Arfon and Ceredigion), but larger northern cities such as Leeds and Liverpool also displayed high indices of dissimilarity. Indices of dissimilarity were again highest for South Asian people in the Pennine towns, rural areas, and cities such as Birmingham and Sheffield. Indices of dissimilarity for Indian people were highest in rural areas, notably in the South West of England and the west of Wales. Pakistani people experienced extreme levels of segregation in coastal and remoter rural districts with small Pakistani populations, but levels of segregation in larger manufacturing cities and towns such as Derby, Rotherham and Oldham were also very high. The highest Index of Dissimilarity values for 'Chinese and Other' people was recorded in rural areas, notably in the Northern Region of England and Wales, but high segregation values also occurred in Birmingham and Pennine cities.

Table 3.17 summarises the change in segregation by district between 1981 and 1991. The left-hand side of the table identifies those districts in which the value of the Index of Dissimilarity for minority ethnic groups taken as a whole decreased most. Clearly, most are rural areas or else represent small manufacturing towns, in which the large index change represents the effect of large percentage changes in the minority population, within a small total. The right-hand side presents the largest increases in the Lieberson index, listing those districts in which the degree of isolation of minority ethnic groups increased most over the decade from 1981-91. Pennine towns are prominent at the top of the ranking. However, this also reveals that the distribution of minority ethnic groups in some of the larger cities, including Birmingham, Leicester, Bradford and Cardiff, became more concentrated and isolated from white people over the decade. This resulted from the rapid increase of the minority population in larger cities, while the white population continued the 'counter-urbanisation' trend of moving away from the cities and larger towns to smaller towns and rural areas.

As was shown earlier in this chapter, the age structure of the minority ethnic group population is such that it is likely to continue to increase at a relatively rapid rate in the medium term, since young people (especially women aged 16-49, the childbearing age range) represent a larger-than-average share of the population. This factor is reinforced by the higher (though declining over time) fertility rates of minority ethnic groups relative to white people. While no official projections have as yet been made, a number of independent projections of the minority ethnic group population of Britain (of varying degrees of sophistication) have been carried out. At the aggregate level, Ballard and Khalra (1994) suggest that the minority ethnic group population will reach a maximum of about 10% of the British population in the middle of the 21st century. It would then decline in size gradually over time, mirroring a fall in the total population, but the minority share of the population would remain fairly constant.

3.16: Local authority districts with largest Indices of Dissimilarity by ethnic group (1991)

All minorities		Black		South Asian		Indian		Pakistani		Chinese and Other	
Oldham	65.5	England and Wales	65.4	Craven	67.7	South Derbyshire	82.5	Craven	74.0	Berwick-upon-Tweed	92.3
East Staffordshire	63.5	Trafford	56.7	East Staffordshire	65.2	Copeland	73.3	Langbaurgh-on-Tees	71.5	Ceredigion	89.7
Burnley	63.3	Suffolk Coastal	53.2	South Derbyshire	60.4	Ceredigion	72.8	North Warwickshire	69.5	Alnwick	88.9
England and Wales	61.6	Leeds	52.1	Oldham	60.2	Barrow-in-Furness	72.6	Breckland	68.8	Hart	81.7
Hyndburn	60.4	Kirklees	50.4	Rotherham	59.1	England and Wales	69.5	East Staffordshire	67.2	Teesdale	78.9
Rochdale	60.3	Selby	48.7	Burnley	57.6	Preseli Pembrokeshire	69.3	Hambleton	67.1	Castle Morpeth	78.9
Bolton	58.9	Arfon	48.3	Langbaurgh-on-Tees	56.9	South Herefordshire	68.4	Ceredigion	66.6	England and Wales	78.4
Rotherham	58.9	Wansbeck	47.7	England and Wales	56.9	Bolton	68.1	Chester-le-Street	65.1	Arfon	77.8
Pendle	58.5	Ceredigion	44.1	Rochdale	56.5	Torridge	67.3	Weymouth and Portland	64.3	Easington	77.4
Birmingham	58.4	Richmondshire	43.6	Calderdale	55.7	Cotswold	66.9	England and Wales	64.2	Birmingham	77.2
Blackburn	58.3	Derwentside	43.5	South Herefordshire	55.1	Tynedale	66.6	Daventry	63.7	Brecknock	77.0
Calderdale	57.8	Liverpool	42.6	Birmingham	55.1	Castle Morpeth	66.1	Derby	63.1	Leeds	77.0
Bradford	57.3	East Staffordshire	42.1	Ceredigion	53.7	Ribble Valley	65.0	Rotherham	62.6	Bradford	76.1
South Derbyshire	57.0	Wycombe	41.9	Bolton	53.6	East Lindsey	64.4	Oldham	62.2	Blackburn	76.1
Ceredigion	55.1	Eden	41.4	Hyndburn	52.5	Montgomeryshire	64.1	Swale	61.7	Newcastle-under-Lyme	75.7
Derby	54.4	Cotswold	41.2	Sheffield	52.2	Blackburn	64.1	Chiltern	61.4	Ynys Mon-Isle of Anglese	75.4

Table 3.17: Largest changes in index values by district (1981-91)

District	Index of Dissimilarity	District	Lieberson index
Allerdale	−23.4	Burnley	−0.093
Forest Heath	−22.9	Oldham	−0.075
South Northamptonshire	−22.8	South Derbyshire	−0.059
North Norfolk	−22.6	Pendle	−0.058
Cherwell	−21.9	Woking	−0.050
Mid-Bedfordshire	−21.5	Peterborough	−0.041
Craven	−21.3	Rochdale	−0.039
South Hams	−18.4	Trafford	−0.036
Wear Valley	−18.3	Hyndburn	−0.033
King's Lynn and West Norfolk	−17.1	Birmingham	−0.030
Derwentside	−17.0	Oadby and Wigston	−0.030
Alnwick	-16.1	Luton	−0.030
Montgomeryshire	−14.7	Leicester	−0.030
Dinefwr	−13.7	England and Wales	−0.028
Suffolk Coastal	−13.5	Arfon	−0.026
Preseli Pembrokeshire	−13.4	Kirklees	-0.025
Huntingdonshire	−13.4	Wycombe	−0.024
Eden	−13.3	North Bedfordshire	−0.023
Carmarthen	−13.2	Newcastle upon Tyne	−0.023
East Yorkshire	−12.5	Three Rivers	−0.023
Sedgefield	−12.4	Bradford	−0.020
West Oxfordshire	−12.0	Wellingborough	−0.020
Hambleton	−11.3	Ceredigion	−0.019
Port Talbot	−11.2	Cardiff	−0.019
Wansbeck	−11.1	Blaby	−0.019

Data availability and future trends

This chapter has presented a profile of the minority ethnic group population of the UK. This picture is incomplete and out of date in places due to the lack of comprehensive data on the ethnic composition of the population between censuses.

Improved information on the ethnic characteristics of the population is of vital importance on a number of grounds. The minority ethnic group population is set to increase substantially, as a result of both indigenous growth and international migration. Projections of the minority ethnic group population are few and far between. However, one of the few recent exercises published – a projection of the population of working age by Metcalf and Forth (2000) – demonstrates that people from minority ethnic groups will form an increasing percentage of the workforce between 1999 and 2009, due to the youthful age structure of minority ethnic groups. Additionally, the analysis presented above has demonstrated the increasing importance of international migration. A percentage of international migrants will be from minority ethnic groups, and it is clear that the growth of some established minority ethnic groups is still being fuelled by international migration.

It is of crucial importance that better information becomes available on the components of minority population growth. Immigration statistics are currently not classified according to ethnic grouping and there is as yet no reliable data on the number and characteristics of emigrants even at the national scale. The current debate on the number of asylum seekers and the potential contribution to meeting employment demand that they and economic migrants could make (as well as their demand for services) is conducted in a vacuum without such data. Moreover, there is almost no information on the geographical distribution of asylum seekers, which is needed to help predict the demand for local services by asylum seekers and adequately fund such services through Standard Spending Assessments. Additionally, a person's ethnic group is not recorded on his or her birth certificate (except in a few pilot exercises); therefore, there is no accurate information on births by ethnic group. There are clearly ethical and philosophical problems in assigning a baby an ethnic group, but the accurate projection of minority populations and the assessment of service needs in the areas of health and education have a pressing need for such information.

The 1990s saw a substantial expansion in ethnic monitoring, in support of equal opportunities policies, and the demand for ethnically classified data has increased dramatically. This will increase due to the effects of recent legislation, such as the 2000 Race Relations (Amendment) Act, which places a duty on public authorities not to discriminate, and government policy moves to try to promote 'community cohesion' as a response to the urban riots of 2001.

As well as collecting more detailed ethnic group data more regularly for more detailed areas, it will also become necessary in future to collect data on a more complete picture of ethnic and cultural identity. It has become clear that religion is an extremely important dimension of minority identity, and it has also been argued that religion is another dimension of discrimination (especially in the case of Islam). Therefore, there is a need for data to measure disadvantage/discrimination by religious group. Even estimating the total number of people from individual religious traditions is currently very difficult. While the census will provide information on religion for the first time, the information cross-tabulated by religion will be very limited. There is still no systematic collection of language data, which is a major problem for the National Health Service and other service providers, who need to know the likely demand from people whose first language is not English, in order to plan the provision of their services. The need for such information is widespread: for example, the private sector (including the minority business sector) needs such information for marketing products and planning media services. Data on language ability and literacy are also of crucial importance for tackling social exclusion, since ability to use English and literacy are poorest in the oldest, most economically disadvantaged and least well sections of the minority ethnic group population.

The 2001 Census of Population will provide the most detailed picture yet of the minority ethnic group population. It will provide crucial information on how this population has changed during an extremely dynamic decade, and provide a benchmark for such monitoring activities. However, central and local government and the Office for National Statistics must be able to follow up the availability of census data with up-to-date data on the ethnic, religious and linguistic composition of the population at a local scale, and to provide projections of the likely trends in the minority population. At present, there are still no plans to collect nationally comprehensive data on the ethnic characteristics of the population between censuses, and the Treasury has recently cancelled plans for a 'mid-term' census in 2006. As the preliminary findings of the 2001 Census trickle out, there are persistent rumours that the 2011 Census will also be cancelled and 'equivalent' data collected through matching individual records. The ethical consequences of explicitly matching sensitive personal data for the first time appear not to have been addressed yet.

Conclusion: issues for the future

This chapter has demonstrated that the minority ethnic group population of the UK has continued to grow rapidly during the 1990s, and has continued to change in character. The original migrant generation and the first minority ethnic groups to become established are now ageing, with increasing numbers of people of retirement age. Other minority groups remain very youthful, and people of mixed parentage are set to increase their share of the younger age groups. The population is becoming more ethnically diverse as new ethnic groups originating in Eastern Europe, Africa and the Middle East increase rapidly in numbers.

The population of the UK is set to increase rapidly in the next few decades, driven mainly by historically high levels of international migration. The minority population will continue to grow relatively rapidly in the first few decades of the 21st century. The extent of growth in the number of people from minority ethnic groups is extremely difficult to forecast, because of the difficulty of estimating the likely future level of migration and its ethnic composition. For example, enlargement of the EU will increase migration from Eastern Europe, possibly providing youthful (and possibly well-qualified) job competition for British people from minority ethnic groups.

As other chapters in this volume demonstrate, there is some evidence that people from minority ethnic groups have made progress in the education system and the labour market during the decade (Owen et al, 2000), with Indian and Chinese people having some of the best examination achievements. Minority ethnic groups are now 'overrepresented' (relative to their share of the population) among university students, and unemployment rates for all ethnic groups are declining. However, progress has not been even across all minority ethnic groups, with black people continuing to underachieve in the education system and Pakistani and Bangladeshi people remaining resolutely at low rankings of economic prosperity.

In recent years, there has been much speculation as to which will be the first 'black' city in Britain, in which the 'minority' population exceeds the white population. Both Birmingham and Leicester have laid claim to this. People from minority ethnic groups already outnumber the white population in some London boroughs, and it is likely that minority population growth will continue to be fastest in London, fuelled by international and internal migration. In London and other cities, it is likely that people from the more economically successful minority ethnic groups will want to move out of the central areas of the cities and into the suburbs and surrounding small towns. This will reduce the rate of increase in the minority populations of these cities and may reduce the level of geographical segregation, but may also result in new forms of inter-ethnic conflict should suburban concentrations of minority ethnic groups become too large.

The 2001 Census will provide vital information on the current position and achievements of minority population during the 1990s, and will show whether (and to what degree) the minority population has decentralised. These baseline data are of vital importance for monitoring equal opportunities and policy implementation, diversity management and service planning. However, the experience of the 1990s is that data for a single year are not adequate and quickly become out of date. There is a continuous requirement for *local* data on the demographics and health of minority ethnic groups, religion and language use, disaggregated by gender, in order that the needs of growing minority communities are assessed and that service providers are aware of them and can plan accordingly.

Existing data sources and data collection methods are no longer adequate. There is a need for the Labour Force Survey to be boosted in areas of minority population, data on demographic rates by ethnic group for local areas to feed into population estimation and projection exercises, and much more systematic ethnic/cultural data collection (via a boosted Home Office Citizenship Survey, for example) linked to monitoring systems.

Notes

[1] Although most of the analyses presented in this chapter will refer to Britain, some of the data are available for the UK only or England and Wales only.

[2] In addition, there is also a continuing in-flow of fiancés and newly married spouses for some (mainly South Asian) ethnic groups.

[3] This includes Eastern Europeans, and probably also Kurds and other Middle Eastern ethnic groups.

[4] Measurement of the Caribbean population is difficult, because a large percentage of the children of this ethnic group are classified as 'Black–Other'. This is due either to the fact that they describe themselves as 'Black–British' or because they are the children of parents from different ethnic groups (nearly 50% of partners of UK-born Caribbean men are white).

FOUR

Ethnic differentials in educational performance

Tariq Modood

Introduction

In Britain, the groups commonly referred to as 'ethnic minorities' did not 'just happen' to migrate and settle recently in Britain, nor do they 'just happen' to suffer racism in Britain. Rather, they are groups whose identity in British society is shaped by migration and 'race' as well as distinctive ethnicities. They are 'racialised ethnicities' (Modood et al, 2002; see also CMEB, 2000). Hence, themes of ethnicity, 'race' and migration shape the choice of groups under discussion here and frame the presentation offered. The groups in question have many features in common with the rest of British society such as the determining character of social class; but our concern here is with what distinguishes them from the rest of society and the interaction of the *differentia* and the commonalities.

From diverse beginnings

The educational qualifications profile of the non-white minority groups at the time of migration and now are quite diverse. Some minority groups are proportionally less qualified than their white peers, and some much more so. This is true when we look at the population as a whole or those who have recently finished their education. Broadly speaking, the ethnic minority population can be divided in two:

- Caribbean, Pakistani and Bangladeshi ethnic groups have lower average qualification levels than white people;
- Indian, African Asian, Chinese and African ethnic groups are more likely than white people to have a higher qualification (A-levels and above).

Among the critical factors in explaining the qualification levels of these groups today is the qualification profile at the time of migration. This can be seen in Figures 4.1 and 4.2. Figure 4.1 shows the proportion among the minority groups without qualifications divided into three 'generations'[1], as well as the qualification levels of white people for the most recent two generations. The source of the data is the Policy Studies Institute (PSI) Fourth National Survey of Ethnic Minorities, which was conducted in 1994[2]. Beginning with the migrant generation, we see that the six minority groups covered by this survey fall into two groupings. The Caribbean, Pakistani and the Bangladeshi groups had high proportions without GCSE or equivalent qualifications (60-75%). On the other hand, only about 45-50% of Indian, African Asian and Chinese migrants were without this level of qualification. All six groups, however, have made educational progress across the generations, though among the Bangladeshi ethnic group it is only among the young that the proportion without qualifications has declined. It was the Caribbean ethnic group (taking men and women together) that initially made the most progress. This meant that second-generation Caribbean men and women were no longer in the same band as the Pakistani and Bangladeshi ethnic groups but had caught up with the other minorities as well as, in fact, their white peers. As native English speakers whose qualifications were from British examination boards, they were the migrant group that one would expect to make most initial progress (although one should note that we are not discussing the acquisition of a high-level qualification but rather the possession of any qualification at all). Moreover, the progress has been made much more by Caribbean women than men. That Caribbean women were more likely than other women to have a qualification certainly contributed to the good overall average achieved by the second-generation Caribbean ethnic group. With today's 20-year-olds, the gender gap has widened to the point that, although exactly the same proportion of white and Caribbean people have no qualifications (25%) – with white women slightly outnumbering men – nearly a third of Caribbean men have no qualification, compared to a sixth of the women.

However, the Pakistani and the Bangladeshi ethnic groups have made the least progress in reducing the proportion within each group of those without qualifications. While among all other groups about 20-25% had no GCSEs, the proportion among these two groups was about double this. What Figure 4.1 shows, then, is this: in terms of having no qualifications, some of the ethnic minority groups were similarly or better placed than their white peers, and some much worse. And, furthermore, this is not something that has just been achieved recently but has been true for some time and partly reflects migrants' starting points. The groups who are worse placed than white people are the Bangladeshi and the Pakistani ethnic groups, as well as Caribbean males.

Figure 4.1, however, does not tell the whole story. What is perhaps more important to look at is not those who have a qualification but those who have *higher* qualifications. Figure 4.2 presents the original profile and generational progress in relation to those who have an A-level or higher qualification. Once again, three migrant groups stand out as well qualified, namely, the Chinese, African Asian and Indian ethnic groups. And three groups were much less well qualified, the Bangladeshi ethnic group especially, but also the Pakistani and

Figure 4.1: Percentage within groups with no GCE or equivalent qualification

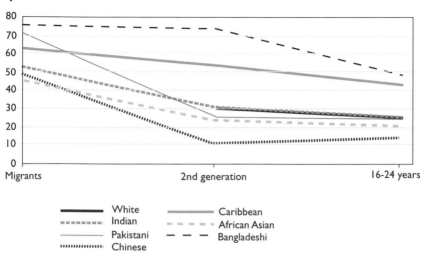

Source: Modood (1998, p 29)

the Caribbean ethnic group. Again, each group (with the exception of the Bangladeshi ethnic group) made progress in the second generation, although the progress of the Pakistani ethnic group was quite minor. Once again, the Caribbean group made the most dramatic progress, although the African Asian ethnic group was the best qualified at this level, considerably ahead of the white group. What Figure 4.2 does not show, however, is that while all other groups (including the Bangladeshi ethnic group) were well represented at degree level, very few Caribbean men or women with higher-level qualifications had degrees (just 2% of the migrants and 7% of the second generation). Many of their higher qualifications were vocational qualifications such as HNCs or nursing qualifications. In contrast, nearly 10% of Pakistani and Bangladeshi migrants and 25% of Indian, African Asian and Chinese migrants had degrees. This meant that some groups such as the Pakistani and Bangladeshi ethnic groups were very internally polarised, with disproportionate numbers of highly qualified and unqualified. However, it did mean that each of these groups had significant proportions of university-educated persons. Therefore, it is not surprising, as we shall see later in this chapter, that these groups have gone on to be well represented in higher education in their second and third generations. That they have not all made equal progress in this regard can partly be correlated to the extent that they had British or overseas qualifications. Thus, the relatively limited progress of second-generation Indian people may be a reflection of the fact that the migrants had a disproportionate number of Indian degrees, compared to the Chinese and African Asian ethnic groups, whose qualifications in the main were from British examination boards and institutions.

Two other important factors should be noted. First, gender differences: male

Figure 4.2: Percentage within groups with A-level or higher qualification

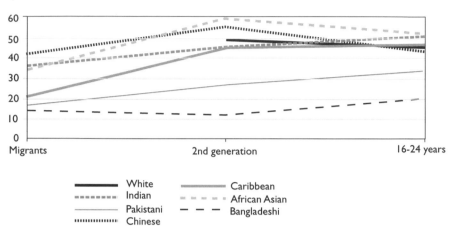

Source: Modood (1998, p 39)

migrants were better qualified than women, especially among the Bangladeshi, Indian and Pakistani ethnic groups. In each group, men were much more likely to have degrees; Caribbean women, however, were and remain much more likely than Caribbean men to have higher qualifications. Second, another factor accounting for the divergent profiles is that, in the pursuit of qualifications, some groups are more vocationally than academically qualified, and so the qualified among them are less likely to have degrees. This is particularly the case among Caribbean and white people, who are much more likely to have a higher vocational qualification than the South Asian ethnic groups, who have a stronger academic orientation.

Schools and young people

In most minority ethnic groups, then, the second and third generations have made significant progress, as have their white peers. Among 16- to 24-year-olds, far fewer are without a qualification than the older generations. The position of Indian, African Asian, Chinese and African men and women is comparable with that of white people, except at degree level where the position of these minorities is distinctly better. Ethnic minority women have made particular progress. By 1995, girls were more likely than boys to achieve five higher-grade GCSEs in each of the principal minority groups. The Pakistani and Bangladeshi ethnic groups, however, continue to have the largest proportions without qualifications, and the position of young Caribbean men is no better than that of their elders.

Data from local education authorities suggest that at the beginning of schooling, and at the time of the first national tests at age seven, the differences between Caribbean and white children are relatively slight, and sometimes in the favour of the Caribbean children. It is the South Asian children, often coming from homes in which English, if spoken at home, is a second or third language, who begin their school careers with low averages. However, they slowly catch up, and in the case of some groups, overtake the white children. The Caribbean children's average steadily drops behind that of the national average (Owen et al, 1999; Richardson and Wood, 1999; Gillborn and Mirza, 2000; Berthoud et al, 2000, p 10).

Explanations of these differences have tended to focus on Caribbean males, who experience very high rates of disciplinary action and exclusion from school (Gillborn and Gipps, 1996, pp 50-3). There is general agreement that they have the most confrontational relations with teachers. Teachers, for their part, report that they feel most threatened and frightened by young Caribbean males. One explanation emphasises teacher racism (Gillborn, 1998; Connolly, 1998). This can be based upon the perceptions of teachers, acquired and fostered through a staff-room culture and through disciplinary problems with previous pupils, that lead to low expectations about the behaviour and work of Caribbean boys, and can lead teachers to interpret certain behaviour more negatively than similar behaviour exhibited by white or Asian males. It might even lead to pre-emptive disciplining (Gillborn, 1990, 1998). There can also be forms of indirect discrimination at play, whereby procedures and organisational arrangements that may have nothing to do with 'race' and ethnicity directly, may nevertheless have disproportionately negative impacts on Caribbean boys. Take setting for example: it is an arrangement that may result in Caribbean boys being disproportionately placed in lower sets and thereby less likely to be prepared for certain exams (Gillborn and Youdell, 2000). (Of course, it is quite possible for an arrangement that negatively impacts upon one minority group to have positive impacts upon another.)

An alternative type of explanation in relation to Caribbean boys emphasises that the high levels of confrontation and disciplining are at least partly due to what the boys bring into school with them (Mac an Ghaill, 1988; Sewell, 1997). It is argued that they draw on a youth or street culture and specifically "on a Black collectivist anti-school ideology, on a pro-consumerism and phallocentrism" (Sewell, 1997, p 108). This culture gives black boys the collective strength to resist racism but it undervalues academic achievement. Indeed, academic aspirations are disparaged as a form of 'acting white', and the living out of this black masculinity inevitably leads to failing to meet the norms of school behaviour. "In this way, a vicious cycle can develop in which what is perceived as a lack of respect from teachers is met by an aggressive response from pupils who in turn are punished for the behaviour" (Pilkington, 1999, p 415).

Aspects of this view are gathering support among the black community, which is concerned with the development of a 'gangsta' culture and the absence of good male role models at home, as well as in schools (Abbot, 2002; Clunis, 2002; Phillips, 2002).

Each explanation may be true to a degree, but the first explanation raises an unnoticed paradox: if racism leads to victims being 'turned off' school and dropping out, why do Asian men and women have such high staying-on rates and make academic progress? While recognising that there are significant differences between the racism experienced by the Caribbean and Asian ethnic groups, as captured in the plural idea of *racisms* (CMEB, 2000, chapter 5), ethnographic research suggests, in ways consistent with surveys, that Asian students experience more frequent and more violent racial harassment from other pupils than do Caribbean students (Gillborn, 1998;Virdee et al, 2000). I am not aware of any research that has studied why this high-level peer racism and bullying does not stop Asian students from persisting with high levels of motivation and performance.

Suffice to say that, as far as I am aware, no convincing explanations exist to fully account for the above differentials. I would like to make two suggestions. First, that the research and policy focus for the past three decades has asked why Caribbean males do not make progress in British schools, rather than why some Asian groups do make progress. Some focus on the latter must surely help us to understand better some of the processes in relation to ethnicity, racism, schooling and attainments. Second, it seems to me that what happens in schools is probably only a small part of a much bigger picture. I return to this issue later in this chapter when I offer some speculation about causal processes.

What cannot be denied is that, in general, ethnic minorities manifest a strong drive for qualifications, and once they begin to acquire qualifications, they seek more. For example, when we look at those with a GCSE or higher qualification who were continuing in (or had returned to) full-time education, we see a degree of minority commitment quite different from that of white people. While a quarter of the qualified 16- to 24-year-old white people were likely to be in full-time education (slightly more for women, slightly less for men), nearly half of women from ethnic minority groups and well over half of the men were in full-time education. The commitment to education is manifest in groups that were not particularly well qualified at the time of migration: qualified Caribbean men and women in this cohort were considerably more likely to be in full-time education than their white peers, and qualified Pakistani/ Bangladeshi men and women had the highest participation rate for each sex in the PSI survey[3].

Some of the high level of minority participation in post-compulsory full-time education is likely to be a reflection of the fact that ethnic minorities used to take longer to achieve their qualifications, but this has since declined. Moreover, white people, especially white men, are more likely to be in work and to be pursuing their further education and training while in work or in training that is linked to work (Drew et al, 1992; Drew, 1995; Hagell and Shaw, 1996). Furthermore, the presence of high rates of youth unemployment, especially among those without qualifications, and the knowledge that ethnic minorities suffer much higher rates of unemployment, may all be thought to

Table 4.1: Proportion of qualified 16- to 24-year-olds in full-time education (%)

	White	Caribbean	Indian/ African Asian	Pakistani/ Bangladeshi	All ethnic minorities
Has O-level or higher and is in full-time education					
Men	21	34	63	71	58
Women	28	40	47	48	46
Weighted count					
Men	163	105	166	105	413
Women	145	137	187	101	471
Unweighted count					
Men	116	48	110	119	293
Women	119	73	124	119	334

Source: PSI Fourth Survey of Ethnic Minorities (Modood et al, 1997, p 76)

add to the explanation of why the ethnic minorities have high staying-on rates.

The evidence is, however, that the ethnic minority youngsters who do – or who are allowed to stay on – do so for positive reasons. A study of 16-year-olds in six inner-city areas also found that minority ethnic individuals were more likely to stay on than white people. Of those that stayed on, 50% wanted to go to university at some point in the future, while less than 20% said that staying on was better than being unemployed (Hagell and Shaw, 1996, p 88). Further analysis of that survey shows that Asian students were no more likely than white students (and Caribbean students little more likely) to say that they stayed on in education because it was better than being unemployed. On the other hand, ethnic minorities were much more likely than white people to say that they wanted to improve their educational qualifications or go to university. The knowledge that qualifications are necessary for getting a (desirable) job may well motivate ethnic minorities more than white people, but it seems to do so positively rather than negatively (Wrench and Qureshi, 1996; Basit, 1997). However, there may be features about schools that ethnic minorities wish to avoid, for they disproportionately transfer from school to further education (FE) colleges to study subjects and for exams that are available at school. Moreover, some minority groups, especially the Caribbean ethnic group, drop out of school at the age of 16 and pick up their studies at FE at a later date (Owen et al, 2000).

Higher education

Thus far, we have seen higher participation rates in post-16 education among the ethnic minorities. It will come as no surprise to learn, then, that, contrary to the claims of most commentators at the time, when admissions to higher education began to be monitored in 1990, ethnic minorities were not underrepresented (Modood, 1993). Moreover, all minority groups, with the possible exception of the Caribbean ethnic group, have increased their share of admissions since then. Ethnic minorities as a whole are about 50% more successful in achieving university entry than white applicants, but not evenly so. More than twice the proportion of 18- to 24-year-old African, Chinese, Asian–Other and Indian students enter university than white students, and no minority group is underrepresented as such (Table 4.2). Some gender differences persist, however, as Caribbean men and Bangladeshi women are underrepresented, but in the latter case there is a trend towards equal or overrepresentation. Otherwise, it is only the white people that are underrepresented in both genders. So, the minority groups, with the exception of Caribbean men, are on different points of an escalator, all moving upwards relative to white students and, in fact, some groups exceeded the government's target of 50% participation by age 30 some years ago.

While some minorities are very well represented in competitive subjects, they are (with the exception of Chinese students) still generally more likely to be in the less prestigious, less well-resourced post-1992 universities. This is especially true of Caribbean students (Modood and Acland, 1998), who are also more likely to be mature students – more than half of Caribbean women students are over 25 years old (Owen et al, 2000; Pathak, 2000) – and part-time students (Owen et al, 2000). Each of these factors has implications for career prospects. A-level scores, subject preferences, preference for local institutions, and type of school or college attended are all factors that explain the concentration of ethnic minority groups (again, with the exception of Chinese students) in the new universities. Nevertheless, a recent analysis shows that, even accounting for these factors, there is a clear institutional effect (Shiner

Table 4.2: Domiciled first year full-time and part-time students (1997-98)

	% in higher education	% 18-24s in higher education	% of 18-24s in Britain	18-24s gender balance in higher education (male – female)
White	84.9	85.2	92.0	48[a] – 52[a]
Indian	4.1	4.7	2.0	51 – 49
Pakistani	2.5	2.7	1.8	56 – 44
Bangladeshi	0.7	0.7	0.7	58 – 42[a]
Chinese	0.9	1.0	0.4	50 – 50
Asian–Other	1.2	1.2	0.4	52 – 48
African	2.1	1.4	0.6	48 – 52
Caribbean	1.3	1.0	0.9	40[a] – 60
Black–Other	0.6	0.5	0.7	38[a] – 62

Note: [a] Denotes underrepresentation.

Source: Higher Education Statistics Agency, 1991 Census and Labour Force Survey, 1999-2000

and Modood, 2002). The analysis shows that lower A-level predictions by schools on UCAS forms do not seem to be a factor. In fact, schools make more generous predictions for ethnic minority candidates, with the most optimistic forecasts made about Black African and Caribbean students, contrary to what one might expect on the basis of the teacher racism we considered earlier (Shiner and Modood, 2002, p 217).

Table 4.3 presents the results of a multivariate analysis, which shows that, comparing similarly qualified candidates and controlling for factors such as public schools, gender and so on, new (post-1992) universities respond more positively than old universities to non-white applicants. Furthermore, within this sector, Chinese, Bangladeshi and Indian candidates appear to be favoured over white candidates: white candidates have a 73% chance of eliciting an offer from a new university, lower than that of their ethnic minority peers. When applying to old universities, however, there is strong evidence that minority candidates face an ethnic penalty. Institutions within this sector are most likely to select white and, to a lesser extent, Chinese candidates from among a group of similarly qualified applicants. Given the much larger proportion of applications from ethnic minority groups, although ethnic minority applicants may be admitted to old universities in reasonable numbers, they generally have to perform better than their white peers in order to secure a place. As the type of institution from which one graduates can make a big difference to one's career prospects, this bias can have serious, long-term implications for ethnic stratification (Shiner and Modood, 2002). It ought to be borne in mind, however, that some ethnic minority groups have a disproportionately large amount of their 18- to 24-year-olds in higher education, and therefore are digging deeper into the natural talent available in that age group. Hence, it is

Table 4.3: Probability of eliciting an initial offer

| | Type of institution applied to | |
	Old	New
White	0.75	0.73
Black–Caribbean	0.65[a]	0.75
Black–African	0.57[a]	0.76
Indian	0.58[a]	0.85[a]
Pakistani	0.57[a]	0.77
Bangladeshi	0.57[a]	0.82[a]
Chinese	0.68[b]	0.83[a]

Notes:
[a] $p = <0.01$
[b] $p = 0.018$
ns = not significant ($p = >0.01$)

For each type of institution, significance tests compare the probability of success for each minority group with that of white people.

Source: Shiner and Modood (2002)

not surprising in itself that a larger proportion of their applicants enter institutions that require lower A-level entry scores. For, were we to compare like with like, the peers of some who enter these universities are white people who are absent from higher education. This does not, however, negate the generalisation that ethnic minorities have to do better than white people to get into older universities, which, therefore, are complicit in an institutional discrimination that hinders and slows down the dismantling of an ethnic stratification.

Some speculation about causes

Besides the factors mentioned above, social class is probably the most powerful one in explaining the educational outcomes discussed here. However, its effect is heavily qualified. It is clearly qualified by gender norms and expectations in different communities, for example, as we see in the contrasting effects among the Bangladeshi and the Caribbean ethnic groups, although, of course, we must not assume that cultural identities that govern gender or other kinds of norms are static. There are both quantitative and qualitative data to show that cultures that until recently might have been portrayed as opposed to the education and employment of women appear now to be producing growing cohorts of highly motivated young women (Ahmad et al, 2003). Other than through a distinctive gender effect, Caribbean ethnicity, however, has a lesser effect than the others on class and sometimes diminishes the class-based likelihood of success (Penn and Scattergood, 1992; Taylor, 1992; Gillborn and Gipps, 1996). The class position of the Pakistani and Bangladeshi ethnic groups is made worse by the fact that, on the whole, they have larger households, and that married women are unlikely to be in paid employment outside the home, resulting in fewer earners and more dependents in a household. South Asian and the Chinese people, however, seem to do better than one might reasonably expect, given their parental class. This can be seen from Table 4.4, which shows university entrants of 1998 by ethnicity, gender and parental social class. It shows an absence of gender difference; unsurprisingly, class is a major factor.

Table 4.4: UCAS entrants by ethnicity, gender and parental social class (1998)

	White		Chinese		Indian		Pakistani		Bangla- deshi		African– Carib- bean[a]		Black– African	
	M	F	M	F	M	F	M	F	M	F	M	F	M	F
Non-manual	67.1	67.4	52.5	52.7	48.5	48.4	36.5	36.1	36.3	35.8	52.1	56.4	51.5	54.8
Manual	25.2	24.6	33.7	33.7	39.5	39.7	39.7	38.2	39.2	38.9	26.9	24.4	20.5	19.3
Unknown[b]	7.7	13.8	13.6	12.1	12.0	23.8	25.8	24.5	25.3	21.0	19.2	28.1	25.9	8.0

[a] Includes Black–Caribbean and Black–Other.
[b] Most parents whose social class UCCA classifies as unknown appear to have been unemployed.
Source: Ballard (1999)

In nearly every group, the offspring from parents with non-manual occupations exceed, sometimes by a large margin, those from parents with manual occupations. This is particularly the case among white people, but is also of considerable magnitude among the Black–African and African-Caribbean ethnic groups. However, it has much less significance for Indians and Chinese, groups in which entrants are almost equally likely to come from non-manual as from other backgrounds, including unemployment. And the conventional class analysis does not hold at all for the Pakistani and Bangladeshi ethnic groups, among which households headed by a manual or unemployed worker supply nearly two thirds of the entrants.

To some extent, one might counter, this was because the South Asian and Chinese entrants' parental social class and educational capital was better than that suggested by their parents' occupations, for their occupational levels were depressed by migration effects and discrimination in the labour market. Due to this racial discrimination, migrants often suffered a downward social mobility on entry into Britain (Modood et al, 1997, pp 141-2). The only jobs open to them were often below their qualification levels and below the social class level they enjoyed prior to their migration. This meant that, not only did many value education more than their white workmates, but they saw it as part of the process of reversing the initial downward mobility, especially in the lives of their children. When we recall the qualification levels of the migrants as presented in Figures 4.1 and 4.2, this argument – that migrants' occupational class in Britain is not reflective of their true class and hence of their attitudes to education – seems to have some plausibility. It is particularly plausible in the case of the African Asian ethnic group, and perhaps also the Indian group, but less so with other groups. In any case, class analysis by itself, even after taking initial downward mobility into account, is incomplete without acknowledging the economic motivation of migrants, the desire to better themselves and especially the prospects for their children. The belief in the value of education in achieving upward mobility and respectability is related to this, as is the strong academic orientation of groups such as the South Asian and the Chinese. The same factors are likely to be operative in the case of the African ethnic groups, who were not included in the PSI survey, but emerged in the 1991 and the 2001 Censuses as the group with the highest proportion of persons with higher qualifications (Owen et al, 1997; Frean, 2003).

It is worth noting here the general sociological claim that there is such a thing as an 'Asian trajectory' or an 'Asian future', which includes social mobility by education, self-employment and progression into the professions (Cross, 1994). The implication is that it is wrong to divide South Asian groups into 'successful' and 'disadvantaged' categories, for the latter are likely only to have less longevity of residence in Britain (measuring families and communities, not just individuals) or to have suffered temporary setbacks (perhaps due to economic restructuring). Today's successful Asians (like the Indians) are yesterday's disadvantaged Asians; today's disadvantaged Asians are the successes of tomorrow. This view probably over-homogenises the South Asian ethnic group, and ignores the differential educational and employment backgrounds at the time of migration of different South Asian groups, as well as the differential degrees of segregation and factors peculiar to Muslims (Modood et al, 1997, pp 146-8). Nevertheless, there may still be something in it and it does have the merit of consistency with some perceivable trends. For example, it is supported by the fact, visible in Table 4.4, that South Asian university entrants are less likely than other groups to come from non-manual backgrounds. More particularly, when we compare the three disadvantaged groups – the Pakistani, Bangladeshi and Caribbean ethnic groups – members of the latter group are much more likely to come from non-manual backgrounds than the other two groups, even though they have a similar manual/non-manual profile in the workforce, at least as regards male workers (Modood et al, 1997, tables 4.10 and 4.13). This does lend some weight to the argument that there is an ambition among South Asians to be university-educated, which is not constrained by class, but on the contrary is seen as integral to social mobility ambitions.

I imagine that ethnic minority parents, especially among the South Asian and Chinese groups, are probably less knowledgeable of the school system and participate less in school activities than their white peers. I also doubt that they spend more time on helping with or discussing schoolwork with their children at home, the content of which will be less familiar to them than to white parents. Yet what they do is to foster high expectations (even to the point of pressuring the children), give encouragement, maintain discipline (such as ensuring that homework is done), send children to and help with supplementary classes and so on. In short, what they give is not a transfer of knowledge and skills but a sense that education is important, that teachers should be obeyed, and that academic success takes priority over other pursuits, especially recreational youth culture.

I would emphasise here that it is not just the parents that are critical factors, but also the wider family and ethnic community, since family aspirations need to be reinforced. Min Zhou's (1997, 2004: forthcoming) work in New York's Chinatown, which uses the concept of ethnicity as social capital, shows how the orientation is reinforced by the whole community in all kinds of ways. One of these is the protection of the children and youth from certain kinds of influences, including street and youth cultures. In contrast, Elijah Anderson's (1994) work brings out the difficulties that African-Americans have in avoiding these anti-scholastic influences (see also Ferguson, 2004: forthcoming). Even where parents from different groups have the same aspirations for their children, they may, quite independently of class, have access to quite different forms of social capital to materialise their aspirations.

Of course material resources are also important. While they relate closely to the class configuration of an ethnic group, it is quite likely that the extent of savings and spending priorities is shaped not just by the availability of resources but also by cultural preferences. These preferences are likely to have a class character, but they will also have a significant ethnic dimension. For example, my guess is that ethnic minority parents spend a larger proportion of their disposable income on education than do white parents. There is no systematic evidence for testing this hypothesis, but perhaps what follows could be offered in its support. The 1998 data on university entrants showed that Indian candidates were slightly more likely than white candidates to have come from independent schools, and that Chinese candidates were twice as likely than white candidates to do so (Ballard, 1999; see also Berthoud et al, 2000, p 82). Bearing in mind that these minority groups still have slightly more children per family than white people (Modood et al, 1997, pp 40-1), and a much higher proportion of children applying to universities on a per capita basis Indian candidates are 2.5 times more likely than white people to be in fee-paying schools, and Chinese candidates five times more so[4]. This amounts to a lot of personal financial investment in educational success, despite the fact that the minority groups still have lower spending power per capita than white people, after one adjusts for pensioner households (Modood et al, 1997). The Pakistani and Bangladeshi ethnic groups do not have the same kind of representation in fee-paying schools. However, the very same argument about ethnic preferences can be made in their case too, when one bears in mind that, despite the fact that four out of every five Pakistani and Bangladeshi households are in poverty (Modood et al, 1997), these groups produce a larger proportion of university entrants than the white population.

The continuing presence of racial discrimination has also meant that non-white persons have been particularly dependent on qualifications for jobs and economic progression, especially as they lacked the social networks (such as those associated with Oxbridge or certain working-class occupations) to help them get on. Hence, each of the kinds of factors that I have been referring to – that is, those that are 'internal' to the group and those that are 'external' – have worked together, interacting with and reinforcing each other, to make qualifications and higher education of more value and urgency to the ethnic minority than to the white population[5].

Persisting/growing polarities

The frameworks favoured by researchers in the 1980s assumed that the African-Caribbean experience would be paradigmatic for children of colour ('black' people). Rather, it is more accurately seen as one strand in a multi-faceted story (Richardson and Wood, 1999). It is clear, nevertheless, that significant polarities exist among the ethnic minority groups and within specific minority groups. No single convincing explanation exists that accounts for both pairs of polar ends. Typically, most researchers focus on and attempt to rationalise only one end of one of the polarities, sometimes proceeding as if their chosen end was the whole story. The most polarised groups – namely the Pakistanis and Bangladeshis – happen to be the ones that were in the news in 2001 (the year of the riots and the start of the 'war against terrorism'[6]). While they continue to be much more likely than all other groups to leave school with no qualifications, it is best to remember before one makes generalisations about the group that in 40% of local education authorities that monitor by ethnic origin, Pakistanis are more likely than white people to attain 5 A*-C GCSEs (Gillborn and Mirza, 2000). Furthermore, on a per capita basis, there are more Pakistani students than white students at university. Caribbean men, too, are a continuing cause of concern, and if they are less polarised than other groups, it is because they are largely absent at the top end of the pole. Any social inclusion policy needs to target 'the truly disadvantaged' but it would be no less a mistake to assume that, in relation to educational attainments, any minority group is homogeneous, than to assume that an explanation of the educational profile of one minority group explains them all[7].

Notes

[1] These three generations are, first, the migrants who came to Britain aged 16+; second, those who came to Britain under the age of 16 and so had some schooling in Britain, or were born in Britain, and were between 25 and 44 years of age at the time of the survey; third, the new generation, those who were aged between 16 and 24, most of whom were born in Britain and had most, if not all, of their education in Britain. Strictly speaking, these are not true 'generations' per se, since there could be an age overlap between the first and second groups, and the years are not evenly spread across the three categories.

[2] The PSI survey covered many topics, including employment, earnings and income, families, housing, health, racial harassment, culture and identity. The survey was based on interviews of about an hour in length, conducted by ethnically matched interviewers, and offered in five South Asian languages and Chinese as well as English. Over 5,000 persons were interviewed from these six groups: Caribbean, Indian, African Asian (people of South Asian descent whose families had spent a generation or more in East Africa), Pakistani, Bangladeshi and Chinese. Additionally, nearly 3,000 white people were interviewed, in order to compare the circumstances of the minorities with that of the ethnic majority. Unfortunately, for reasons of costs and logistics, Africans were not included in the survey. Further details on all aspects of the survey are available in Modood et al (1997).

[3] Other data suggest that the African ethnic groups have the highest participation rate of all groups (Berthoud et al, 2000, p 9).

[4] It needs to be borne in mind, therefore, that the widening access policies in some prestigious universities that aim to reduce the proportion of entrants from fee-paying schools, if successful, should lower the proportion of Chinese and Indian candidates admitted to those universities while increasing that of other minority groups. Interestingly, taking the higher education sector as a whole, it has been found that after controlling for A-level scores and a number of other factors, attending an independent school slightly reduced a candidate's chance of admission (Shiner and Modood, 2002, p 229, n 8).

---

[5] Whether this investment in education has paid dividends in terms of jobs and incomes is a complex question, but it seems not to have done so for at least the African group (Berthoud, 1999, 2000a).

[6] These events precipitated a moral panic about 'faith schools' without any evidence being offered that anyone involved in the riots or any Islamist organisation had been to a 'faith school'.

[7] More detailed support for the arguments in this chapter can be found in Modood et al (1997, chapter 3) and in Modood (1998).

FIVE

Changing patterns of ethnic disadvantage in employment

David Mason

Introduction

In Chapter Four, we saw that significant changes were occurring in the experiences of minority ethnic groups in the education system. The pattern of upward mobility revealed in that chapter runs counter to many taken-for-granted assumptions, including those surrounding the supposed persistence of 'educational underachievement' (see Mason, 2000, pp 62-78). This is not to deny, of course, that significant inequalities persist. They relate to two key themes of this book: the increasingly differentiated experiences of Britain's minority ethnic citizens and the persistence of disadvantage relative to the 'white' population.

It is arguable that labour market position and employment status are central issues in understanding differences in the experiences of Britain's minority ethnic groups. This is because the resources that derive from employment are keys to accessing a range of other desired goods and services. The extent to which this is so is illustrated by the analyses of both health and housing presented in Chapters Six and Seven of this volume. It is no surprise then, to find that members of minority ethnic groups identify labour market success as key aspects of their life strategies. In this context, Modood's analysis in Chapter Four emphasised the extent to which the apparent drive by young minority ethnic people to acquire qualifications is a response to the labour market experiences of their parents and their own perceptions of the patterning of opportunities open to them. In this regard, education can be seen, in some respects, as representing an investment in labour market futures. As we shall see, the patterning of that investment is, to some degree, reflected in the labour market experience of different groups. Yet at the same time, it is clear that the returns on that investment are not equivalent for all groups. There is, as we shall see, evidence of a continuing ethnic penalty that operates notwithstanding substantial occupational mobility among members of at least some groups. This penalty relates not only to the kinds of jobs that can be accessed. It also has implications for financial returns to employment in the form of incomes.

This last point is crucial because, as we shall see, employment patterns interact with other aspects of individual and family strategies, shaping significant differences between the household incomes of different groups. Moreover, as Chapter Nine of this volume makes clear, there are other dimensions to individual and collective well-being, associated with a sense of full citizenship, that do not simply vary with socioeconomic status.

In the remainder of this chapter we first review some long-standing patterns that characterise the labour market positions of minority ethnic groups. We then examine the evidence that suggests that some groups are experiencing significant upward occupational mobility. Finally, we set these trends in the context of evidence of a continuing ethnic penalty, before going on to note that, even where it occurs, labour market success may not have the same beneficial consequences for members of all groups in terms of material well-being.

Settlement patterns and employment

The data presented in Chapter Three clearly show how the circumstances in which postwar migrants came to Britain had enduring implications for their employment opportunities. Attracted by, and often recruited to fill, specific vacancies in areas of labour shortage – notably in the least desirable jobs at the bottom of the labour market – the new migrants tended to concentrate in urban conurbations where such jobs were to be found. As Owen's analysis in Chapter Three shows, their descendants have tended to continue to live in these broad areas of initial settlement. Indeed, there has been relatively little geographical expansion. This, of course, has had direct effects on the range of employment opportunities which it has been possible to access (see the discussion in Owen and Green, 1992, 2000), and this in turn helps to account for the apparent persistence of a relatively stable pattern of disadvantage, at least until recently.

Research conducted through the 1960s, 1970s and 1980s (Daniel, 1968; Smith, 1976; Brown, 1984) revealed a pattern of continuing disadvantage with people from minority ethnic groups clustered in particular industries and occupations and overrepresented in semi-skilled and unskilled jobs. In addition, there has been a persistent pattern of exclusion altogether from the labour market, with members of minority ethnic groups experiencing consistently lower participation rates and higher rates of unemployment than their white counterparts. As we shall see, there is evidence, particularly following the de-industrialisation of the 1980s, of new patterns emerging and of more recent patterns of upward occupational mobility. However, each of these must be set in the context of distinct patterns of labour market exclusion.

Labour market inclusion and exclusion

The percentage of men of working age active in the labour market is highest for the white, Indian and Caribbean ethnic groups (Table 5.1)[1]. Bangladeshi,

Pakistani and Other–Mixed men are least likely to be economically active. The pattern for women is similar, but the percentages active in the labour market are lower. Around four fifths of white men, but only two thirds of men from minority ethnic groups, are in employment, while 70.3% of white women, but only half of women from minority ethnic groups, are in employment. Only two thirds of Caribbean men are in work, a slightly higher percentage than for Black–African men, but three quarters of Indian men are in work. The employment rate for Caribbean women is similar to that of men, but that for Black–African women is rather lower. Indian women have the highest employment rate among minority ethnic groups other than Caribbean people, but employment rates for Pakistani and Bangladeshi women are extremely low.

There are some important differences between groups that are concealed by these figures. In particular, the younger age profiles of the minority ethnic populations means that a larger proportion of those who are economically inactive are of working age when compared with the white population. In addition, there are significant gender variations between groups. Mirza (1992, p 164) has suggested that the patterns of labour market participation characteristic of African-Caribbean women reflect the specific cultural construction of femininity in communities where gender roles are more equal, and male and female roles characterised by a relative autonomy (see also Leslie et al, 1998, p 499). Similarly, the relatively low participation rates of women from some Asian groups probably reflect "differences in culture concerning the role of women in home-making and child-rearing" (Jones, 1993, pp 63-4).

Labour market participation data, of course, conceal important differences between full- and part-time working. Part-time employment is dominated by women, who account for nearly 90% of such employees. However, a significantly higher proportion of white women in paid employment work part-time than do those of minority ethnic origin. Moreover, the feminisation of part-time working is less marked among ethnic minorities than among white people, with particularly high levels of part-time working among men of Bangladeshi, Pakistani, and Black–African origin. As Owen (1993, pp 3-4) has pointed out, the relatively high proportion of men among part-time workers in the Bangladeshi and Pakistani groups may, in part, be a consequence of low rates of labour market participation among women from these groups. However, it may also reflect the overrepresentation of men from minority ethnic groups in insecure and poorly paid jobs in what is sometimes called the secondary labour market, where the growth in part-time as well as casualised employment has been significant.

Table 5.1 shows that the minority unemployment rate is twice the white rate for men and three times the white rate for women. This pattern is long-standing, and dates back to the 1980s at least, although there are year-on-year variations (Smith, 1976; Smith 1981; Brown, 1984; Jones, 1993). Moreover, Jones (1993, p 112) argues that unemployment among people from minority ethnic groups is "hyper-cyclical"; that is, in times of recession, the minority

Table 5.1: Economic activity by ethnic group for persons of working age (1998-2000)

	Men				Women			
	Economic activity rate (%)	Employment rate (%)	Unemployment rate (%)	All of working age	Economic activity rate (%)	Employment rate (%)	Unemployment rate (%)	All of working age
White	85.1	79.9	6.1	17,760,674	73.9	70.3	4.9	16,066,867
Minority ethnic groups	**76.4**	**66.2**	**13.4**	**1,209,652**	**55.8**	**49.0**	**12.2**	**1,189,705**
Black	78.4	65.1	16.9	346,110	67.1	57.6	14.1	375,554
Caribbean	80.0	66.3	17.2	220,130	71.3	62.1	12.9	246,745
Black–Caribbean	80.2	67.8	15.5	157,961	72.7	64.4	11.3	173,377
Black–Mixed	78.7	62.7	20.3	31,334	65.4	54.5	16.7	38,298
Black–Other (non-mixed)	80.6	62.5	22.4	30,835	70.7	58.8	16.9	35,070
Black–African	75.4	63.0	16.5	125,980	59.0	49.1	16.8	128,809
South Asian	76.9	67.6	12.0	609,970	47.9	42.4	11.5	552,611
Indian	81.4	74.9	8.0	337,049	63.0	58.0	7.9	308,696
Pakistani	72.8	60.8	16.4	196,920	31.2	25.2	19.2	180,338
Bangladeshi	67.2	53.1	20.9	76,001	22.0	15.4	29.8	63,576
Chinese and Other	72.6	64.1	11.8	253,573	56.5	50.6	10.5	261,540
Chinese	64.4	58.4	9.4	562,88	57.7	53.3	7.6	59,911
Other–Asian (non-mixed)	76.9	70.1	8.9	77,705	55.3	49.6	10.4	86,437
Other–Other (non-mixed)	68.4	56.2	17.9	71,392	48.5	41.5	14.3	58,461
Other–Mixed	81.5	72.6	10.9	48189	65.1	58.4	10.2	56731
All ethnic groups	**84.6**	**79.1**	**6.5**	**18,970,327**	**72.6**	**68.8**	**5.3**	**17,256,572**

Note: Counts of less than 3,000 have been suppressed.

Source: Labour Force Survey

ethnic unemployment rate rises faster than that of white people, while in times of recovery, it falls more rapidly. Once again, however, there are differences between groups. The hyper-cyclical effect appears to be strongest for Caribbeans and Africans and weakest for Pakistanis and Bangladeshis (Berthoud, 2000a).

Overall, unemployment rates for Caribbean and Black–African men are similar, at about a sixth of those that are economically active. The unemployment rate for Caribbean women is somewhat lower. Among people from minority ethnic groups, unemployment rates are highest for the Bangladeshi, Pakistani and Black–Other ethnic groups, and lowest for the Indian and Chinese ethnic groups. Even among these groups, however, the rates for men are a third or more higher than the white rate for men and almost double for women. Interesting, Leslie et al (1998, p 490) have argued that "Indians have characteristics that should lead to a lower rate of unemployment (compared with white people) than to the higher rates actually observed".

It is also important to note that unemployment rates for 16- to 24-year-olds are consistently higher than those for the economically active as a whole (Jones, 1993, p 113; Owen, 1993, p 8; Leslie et al, 1998, p 490). This is of considerable importance, given the relatively younger age structure of minority ethnic groups. Moreover, similar ethnically structured differentials can be identified among young people as among the economically active as a whole. It appears that only among men of African Asian origin (Jones, 1993, p 113) and among Chinese men (Owen, 1993, p 7) are unemployment rates as low as those for white people (compare Modood, 1997b, pp 88-93). Moreover, the true position may also be masked by the higher post-compulsory educational participation of minority ethnic young people.

There is some evidence that unemployment rates vary between different areas of the country. A number of urban locations in the north of England and the Midlands with high levels of unemployment are also areas of substantial minority ethnic residence. As a result, the local patterns of variation between white people and those from minority ethnic groups, as well as between members of different groups, diverge from the overall national pattern. The precise character of these variations is too complex to be dealt with here (but see Jones, 1993; Owen, 1993). However, we can note that levels of minority ethnic unemployment tend to be consistently higher than the white rate. Differences are greater outside Greater London, and, outside this area, even groups such as African Asians are likely to experience higher unemployment than white people (Jones, 1993, pp 113-14; Modood, 1997b, pp 88-93). Having said this, it is not clear that geographical distribution itself can be said to account for differences between white and minority unemployment rates (Fieldhouse and Gould, 1998).

Occupation and job levels

We noted above that it has long been a commonplace supported by data from a series of studies dating back to the 1960s that members of minority ethnic groups have been employed in less skilled jobs, at lower job levels than white people and that they have been concentrated in particular industrial sectors (Daniel, 1968; Smith, 1976; Brown, 1984). More recent data such as Jones's (1993) reanalysis of the Labour Force Survey (LFS) for 1988, 1989 and 1990, and the fourth Policy Studies Institute (PSI) survey (Modood, 1997b) have, however, begun to suggest that the position is becoming more complex as the experience of members of different groups has begun to diverge.

Table 5.2 suggests that male members of some minority ethnic groups are beginning to experience employment patterns increasingly similar to those of white men. This is true of African Asian, Chinese and, to a slightly lesser extent, Indian men, where the proportions approximate or exceed the proportions of white workers in each of the top two categories. However, these figures conceal important variations since, although African Asian and Chinese men are more likely to be professional workers than white men, they are considerably less likely to be represented among senior managers in large enterprises. Among those of Caribbean, Bangladeshi and Pakistani descent, there is much less evidence of progress in the top category (although there is some convergence in the 'intermediate and junior non-manual' category). Bangladeshi men in particular, 53% of whom are in semi-skilled manual occupations, remain concentrated in the lower echelons of the labour market. In addition, we should note that some groups display marked bipolarity. Thus,

Table 5.2: Job levels of men

Socioeconomic group	White	Carib-bean	Indian	African Asian	Pakis-tani	Bang-ladeshi	Chinese
Professional/managers/ employers	30	14	25	30	19	18	46
Employers and managers (large establishments)	11	5	5	3	3	0	6
Employers and managers (small establishments)	11	4	11	14	12	16	23
Professional workers	8	6	9	14	4	2	17
Intermediate and junior non-manual	18	19	20	24	13	19	17
Skilled manual and foremen	36	39	31	30	46	7	14
Semi-skilled manual	11	22	16	12	18	53	12
Unskilled manual	3	6	5	2	3	3	5
Armed forces or N/A	2	0	3	2	2	0	5
Non-manual	48	33	45	54	32	37	63
Manual	50	67	52	44	67	63	31
Weighted count	789	365	349	296	182	61	127
Unweighted count	713	258	356	264	258	112	71

Column percentages

Source: Modood et al (1997)

both Indian and Chinese men are found in large numbers in both the highest and the lowest job categories. Jones (1993, p 70[2]) argues:

> This may suggest that men from these two groups enter a relatively narrow range of occupations, either at the top or bottom end of the job market.

Table 5.3 presents comparable data for women. It shows that women of all groups are less likely than men to be in the top category and, for all groups, the largest concentrations are to be found in the 'intermediate' and 'junior non-manual' categories, followed by 'semi-skilled manual'. This finding matches that of the 1982 PSI survey (Brown, 1984) and Jones's (1993) reanalysis of LFS data. Each of these studies offered a similar explanation. This is that women are already disadvantaged in the labour market relative to men and that, as a result, there is limited scope for an additional disadvantage arising from ethnicity (Jones, 1993, p 71). Despite detailed variations between groups, therefore, there is some evidence that:

> ... gender divisions in the labour market may be stronger and more deeply rooted than differences due to race and ethnicity. (Modood, 1997b, p 104; see also Iganski and Payne, 1996)

So far as distribution between employment sectors is concerned, the data from the LFS reflect both continuity with, and some changes in, the previously established pattern of concentration of the ethnic minority population in

Table 5.3: Job levels of women

Socioeconomic group			*Column percentages*			
	White	Caribbean	Indian	African Asian	Pakistani	Chinese
Professional, managerial and employers	16	5	11	12	12	30
Intermediate non-manual	21	28	14	14	29	23
Junior non-manual	33	36	33	49	23	23
Skilled manual and foremen	7	4	11	7	9	13
Semi-skilled manual	18	20	27	16	22	9
Unskilled manual	4	6	4	1	4	2
Armed forces/ inadequately described/not stated	0	1	1	1	0	0
Non-manual	*70*	*69*	*58*	*75*	*64*	*76*
Manual	*29*	*30*	*42*	*24*	*35*	*24*
Weighted count	*734*	*452*	*275*	*196*	*60*	*120*
Unweighted count	*696*	*336*	*260*	*164*	*64*	*63*

Source: Modood et al (1997)

particular employment sectors. This concentration reflects to some degree patterns of settlement and demand for labour at the time of initial settlement (see Chapters Four and Five of this volume). However, major economy-wide changes in the 1980s associated with the decline in manufacturing employment and the growth of the service sector have led to significant changes for members of all groups. It might be thought that, given their patterns of initial settlement and their concentration in semi-skilled and unskilled manual occupations, the descendants of New Commonwealth migrants to Britain would have fared rather badly in these transformations. In fact, the evidence suggests that, continued disadvantage and exclusion notwithstanding, minority ethnic groups were not disproportionately negatively affected (Iganski and Payne, 1999).

The LFS data for 1988, 1989 and 1990 suggest that the largest proportions of all groups, including white employees, are now to be found in distribution, hotels, catering and repairs. Within this broad pattern, people of South Asian origin are rather more likely than white people to be employed in retail distribution, while those of Chinese and Bangladeshi origin are markedly more likely than white people to work in hotels and catering. Pakistani and Bangladeshi men are particularly likely to be found in the textile and footwear sectors. Among Afro-Caribbeans, there is a relatively high concentration of employees in transport and communication. Afro-Caribbean men are well represented in construction and women in the hospital and healthcare sectors. There is a marked concentration of women of all groups in the service sector, reflecting the general pattern of segregation of women in employment (Jones, 1993, pp 66-8; compare Rees, 1992).

As we have seen, some caution has to be exercised in interpreting the data that are available. Apparently similar proportions of groups in the same occupational category may conceal important differences in status, in the kinds of enterprise worked in, or in the working conditions enjoyed by members of different groups. Thus, it appears that even successful members of minority ethnic groups may have greater difficulty in accessing high-status positions in major companies. This in turn may help to explain the enthusiasm of minority ethnic students for the professions where opportunities exist for the establishment of independent practices. A good example is the legal sector, where minority ethnic groups are increasingly overrepresented among students registering with the Law Society, while remaining underrepresented in large firms of solicitors and in the higher reaches of the legal profession. For example, in April 1998, only 17 of 974 Queen's Counsel (QCs) were of minority ethnic origin, compared with 8.5% of qualified barristers in independent practice and 25% of students enrolling on the Bar Vocational Course in October 1997. Among solicitors, 8.2% on the Roll in England and Wales were of minority ethnic descent compared with 14.9% of those admitted to the profession in 1996-97 (Home Office, 1998, pp 37-8).

These figures are, of course, consistent with increasing recruitment of minority ethnic personnel and, other things being equal, would lead us to expect increasing numbers at higher levels in these professions in future years. Such a pattern would also be consistent with the evidence about the aspirations of minority ethnic young people and known patterns of upward occupational mobility. However, there is still evidence that minority ethnic students find it more difficult to secure trainee positions in the larger and better-paying solicitors' firms – in part because such firms recruit disproportionately from pre-1992 universities where minority ethnic students are underrepresented (Rolfe and Anderson, 2002). Having said this, there is also evidence, following recent initiatives on the recruitment of judges, of increasing success in opening up the higher levels of the profession to minority ethnic groups (Lord Chancellor's Department, 2002).

Another complicating factor in assessing the effects of occupational placement is the question of earnings and hours of work. Brown's (1984) study found that minority ethnic employees had significantly lower earnings than their white counterparts. A number of later studies suggested that this pattern continued into the late 1980s and 1990s (McCormick, 1986; Leicester City Council, 1990; Pirani et al, 1992). This finding is further confirmed by the results of the fourth PSI survey (Modood, 1997b). These reveal, however, marked differences between groups, with African Asian and Chinese men increasingly approximating white rates. Caribbean rates are slightly lower, while Indian, Pakistani and Bangladeshi earnings (in descending order) all fall significantly behind. Among women, there is much less variation with all groups except Bangladeshi women outperforming white women. We must note, however, that these figures are affected by low rates of labour market participation among some groups and by differential patterns of full- and part-time employment[3].

We should note that earnings may be significantly affected by hours worked. In this connection, it is important to note that Brown's study (1984) indicated that members of minority ethnic groups were much more likely than white people to work shifts and that, when this was taken into account, ethnic differentials in earnings were larger than they at first appeared. Jones's (1993) analysis of LFS data for the late 1980s reveals that this difference in the likelihood that members of different groups would work shifts had been maintained to some degree. Pakistani male workers were significantly more likely than others to be working shifts. Among women, those of African-Caribbean origin were the most likely to be engaged in shiftwork. However, what is interesting is that this tendency to work shifts declined with age, suggesting according to Jones that younger people were "not following the older generations into the kinds of jobs which involve shiftwork" (1993, p 75). Whether this reflects choice, employer preference, or the changing structure of employment opportunities is less clear. Given the findings of earlier research, it also raises the question of the likely effect on earnings.

Understanding change: continuity, blip or trend?

There appears to be a growing consensus that, after a period of two decades or so in which ethnic inequalities in the labour market appeared to be relatively intractable, the 1990s saw a process of convergence. As economic change has proceeded, both white people and members of minority ethnic groups appear to have moved into new, and more similar, patterns of labour market experience (compare Iganski and Payne, 1999). As we have seen, the evidence on which this prognosis is based is by no means unambiguous. Debates continue about how to interpret those differences that persist, both between whites and minority ethnic groups and among those groups themselves. Moreover, there are methodological questions about whether the categories in terms of which the data are gathered and organised might not conceal continuing disadvantage. Nevertheless, the studies discussed so far (Jones, 1993; Modood, 1997b) do suggest that (especially male) members of some groups have been experiencing significant upward mobility, with evidence of a high degree of convergence between white people and at least some minority ethnic groups. Moreover, some recent evidence also suggests that these patterns of upward occupational mobility are being matched by a diminution in earnings differentials (Leslie et al, 1998, pp 489, 503-4). As Leslie et al's study (1998) shows, however, it is necessary to bear in mind that the occupational achievements of those in work must be set in the context of continuing disproportionate levels of exclusion altogether from the labour market. Here there is much less evidence of change. We might also note that, to the extent that members of some groups have also made great strides in self-employment, some of the upward mobility experienced by other members of the same groups may well represent a degree of internal segregation of the labour market on ethnic lines.

This model of continuity and change that associates upward mobility with a step change in the 1990s, the reality and robustness of which is open to question, has recently been challenged by Iganksi and Payne (1996) and Iganski et al (2001). Using longitudinal analyses of LFS and Census data dating back to the 1960s, they question whether the evidence supports the idea that long-term cumulative disadvantage has only recently, and conditionally, been interrupted. Instead, Iganski and Payne (1996) argue that a longer-term trend can be discerned in which, in terms of their membership of the Registrar General's socioeconomic categories, minority ethnic groups made steady progress relative to whites between 1966 and 1991. Most importantly, they suggest that even those groups that appear to have been most disadvantaged – Pakistanis and Bangladeshis – also advanced steadily from a generally less favourable starting point. In a more recent paper, Iganski et al (2001) have extended this analysis into the early 21st century by analysing LFS data for 1999 and the first quarter of 2000. They argue that this analysis confirms earlier trends and provides confirmation of the robustness of upward occupational mobility. In particular, they challenge the claim that minority ethnic progress has been limited to the lower echelons of higher labour market positions, claiming that their data show that minority ethnic groups are making slow but steady progress into higher-level positions. They also argue that age-related patterns appear to confirm these trends.

> The younger male cohort has a greater occupational achievement, and a lower 'ethnic gap', than their elders. Newer entrants to the labour force are better able to exploit new kinds of occupational opportunity, whereas older workers in all ethnic groups are more likely to remain trapped in their pre-existing career paths. Where those career paths reflect ethnic disadvantage, this falls more heavily on first generation migrants. (Iganski et al, 2001, pp 198-9)

These observations appear to be consistent with the other trends described and would, if confirmed, lend strength to an optimistic prognosis for greater ethnic equity in the labour market. They are also consistent with the evidence about educational participation and the demonstrable general significance of qualifications in securing employment (Heath and McMahon, 2000). We should note, however, that they are not confirmed by other analyses utilising the LFS (Blackaby et al, 2002).

In setting out their thesis, Iganski and his colleagues acknowledge that the progress they discern in terms of socioeconomic group placement is not matched in the area of unemployment. This, as we have already seen, resists the kinds of changes identifiable elsewhere, for example in relation to earnings. Leslie et al (1998, p 489) argue that this may well be because discrimination with respect to earnings is more visible and hence more open to challenge than the process of exclusion from jobs altogether. Iganski and Payne (1996) also acknowledge that their account is not inconsistent with continued discrimination. This, of course, raises an interesting possibility – namely that, in the absence of discrimination, minority ethnic progress in the labour market might have been even more significant than they argue it already is. In order to address this question, we need to consider how we might explain the ethnic differences that can still be discerned in the labour market.

Explaining ethnic disadvantage in employment

A variety of explanations have been offered for the disadvantage suffered by members of minority ethnic groups in the labour market. Some of the most commonly expressed locate the problem in the character of minority group job seekers. Such explanations draw heavily upon assimilationist assumptions that are widely encountered in explanations of migratory labour. In particular, it is sometimes claimed that migration itself is associated with disadvantage, with recent migrants experiencing greater labour market exclusion than those longer settled, or the second and third generations. Berthoud's (2000a, pp 397-8) analysis, however, has shown not only that migration does not adequately explain ethnic disadvantage, but that its effects appear to differ dramatically between groups. His data appear to show that, among Caribbeans, more recent migrants actually fare better than the longer settled; a finding that is directly opposite to the situation of Pakistanis and Bangladeshis.

It is sometimes argued that high rates of unemployment and low job levels can be accounted for by inadequate English language skills. There is indeed some evidence that those who have poorer English experience more difficulties in the labour market (Brown, 1984, pp 128-49). The fourth PSI survey suggests that both age and length of residence correlate with fluency in English, although it also reveals other sources of variation between members of different groups and between men and women (Modood, 1997a, pp 60-3). However, even if language skills play some part in employment placement, they cannot easily account for the disadvantage experienced by that increasingly large part of the minority ethnic population that was born and educated in the UK. Moreover, it is likely that they are of most use in explaining differences in the lower echelons of the labour market where, incidentally, qualification levels are likely to be of least significance[4].

Another commonly encountered explanation is that minority ethnic workers suffer from skill or qualification deficits when compared with their white counterparts. This argument is often linked to supposed educational 'underachievement'. Once again, there are difficulties with this account. While low levels of qualification are likely to confer disadvantages in the labour market, a number of studies have shown that, when qualifications are controlled for, minority ethnic workers are more likely to be unemployed or in lower job levels than their white counterparts (Smith, 1976; Brown, 1984; Jones, 1993; Berthoud, 2000a; Blackaby et al, 2002). Although the patterns are complex and reveal significant variations, both between groups and between different types of work (Modood, 1997b, pp 91-106; Berthoud, 2000a), there is a consistent message that the returns to education for minority ethnic groups are lower than they might reasonably expect. Even the Indians, who experience a rate of return only slightly lower than whites, do not get full benefit from their investment. This suggests that, while the drive for qualifications noted in Chapter Four of this volume can be rational for some groups, others, such as Africans (Berthoud, 2000a, p 412), continued to fair badly despite high levels of educational qualification.

Other commonly encountered explanations include the effects of family formation (Berthoud, 2000a) and the consequences of differential geographical location (Fieldhouse and Gould, 1998; Owen and Green, 2000). Each can be said to account for some part of the disadvantage suffered by minority ethnic groups. However, there is considerable evidence to suggest that, when such variables are controlled for, there remains a residue of disadvantage and exclusion that cannot be so easily explained. As a result, it is difficult to avoid the conclusion that, despite 35 years of 'race relations' legislation, discrimination continues to play a significant part in the labour market placement of minority ethnic groups.

In this context, it is interesting to note that the fourth PSI survey found that a large majority of all respondents believed that discrimination was widespread.

Indeed, white respondents were the most likely to hold such a view (Modood, 1997b, pp 129-35). This belief is consistent with the findings of an overwhelming body of research evidence that has demonstrated the operation of direct, and apparently intentional, discrimination in employment selection decisions (Daniel, 1968; Hubbock and Carter, 1980; NACAB, 1984; Brown and Gay, 1985). A common method has been to submit job applications from candidates matched in every way except ethnic origin. Using methods such as this, Brown and Gay (1985) revealed continuing systematic discrimination, despite the many years of race relations legislation. Thus, although a substantial number of employers appeared to treat all candidates equally, an equally large number appeared to discriminate. In some cases, Asian applicants were treated more favourably than those of African-Caribbean origin; in others the reverse was true. Overall, however, the researchers found that, while 90% of white applicants were successful, only 63% of Asian and African-Caribbean applicants received positive responses. In other words, white applicants were more than 30% more likely to be treated favourably than those of minority ethnic origin (Brown and Gay, 1985, pp 13-17). The results showed no statistically significant differences in the rate of discrimination between men and women or between older and younger applicants (Brown and Gay, 1985, p 19). Moreover, when compared with the results of earlier studies dating back to the early 1970s, the researchers found no evidence of a diminution in the level of racial discrimination (Brown and Gay, 1985, pp 25-9). Brown and Gay concluded that a major reason for the persistence of discrimination, despite two race relations acts, was that employers were very unlikely to be caught in the act of discrimination (1985, p 33).

Research of this kind, capable of uncovering clear evidence of discrimination, has become less common in recent years. One example (Noon, 1993), conducted some 10 years ago, concerned research into the fate of speculative employment inquiries made to some of Britain's major companies. It has direct implications for the explanations examined above. Matched letters of inquiry were sent to personnel managers at the top 100 UK companies identified from the Times 1,000 Index. The letters were signed by fictitious applicants called Evans and Patel. They were presented as MBA students who were about to qualify and who already had relevant experience. The research compared both the frequencies of responses sent to the two applicants and their quality in terms of the assistance and encouragement offered. It found that, overall, companies were more helpful and encouraging to white candidates. Those with equal opportunities statements in their annual reports were generally more likely to treat both candidates the same. However, 48% of such companies did not treat each candidate equally and, where they did not do so, they favoured the white candidate in proportions greater than those companies without statements. As a result, Noon (1993) argued that his results suggested that discrimination was taking place even in companies ostensibly sensitive to equal opportunities. In this case, we can readily see why the returns to investment in education might vary systematically between groups.

These studies reveal the existence of continuing, apparently direct and deliberate, discrimination. An equally serious problem is posed, however, by what is sometimes called indirect discrimination; that is, where selection criteria are applied equally to everyone but where they are such that they disproportionately affect members of particular groups. A good example is where dress requirements are imposed with which members of some groups, for religious or other reasons, cannot comply, and where the requirements concerned are not necessary for the completion of the occupational task. Indirect discrimination may be deliberate but it is also frequently unintentional and unrecognised. Many of the ordinary, routine, taken-for-granted aspects of the recruitment process and the labour market may give rise to indirect discrimination. Jenkins (1986) has argued that many selection decisions are based not on whether candidates have the right qualifications for the job but on whether they are thought to be likely to 'fit in' to the workplace without causing any trouble. Such judgements are applied equally to each applicant regardless of ethnicity. They become discriminatory when they are consciously or unconsciously informed by stereotypes that managers hold of minority ethnic groups. Jenkins's research revealed, as have other studies (such as Jewson et al, 1990), that negative stereotypes were widespread among managers responsible for recruitment decisions. Although they can operate in the context of recruitment to almost any occupation, it is likely that the significance of these kinds of judgements is greater in respect of those jobs for which particular qualifications are not required.

A recent study of recruitment to nursing and midwifery (Iganski and Mason, 2002) also identified the presence of widespread stereotypes of minority ethnic groups among those responsible for recruitment and selection. Interestingly, these stereotypes often concentrated on the supposed occupational preferences of different groups. Thus, it was often argued that Asian minority ethnic groups exhibited cultural prohibitions on certain kinds of bodily and other contact. This was then invoked as an explanation for the organisation's lack of success in improving the representation of the groups in question. In the process, the organisation absolved itself from responsibility for the situation and, thus, from the need to develop policies and practices to address the shortfall. Even where such recruitment was taking place, however, there was consistent evidence of differential selection outcomes operating to the disadvantage of minority ethnic groups. The authors concluded that most of this occurred at the shortlisting stage, where a lack of system opened up opportunities for capricious decision making informed by stereotyped judgements (Iganski and Mason, 2001).

There is also evidence that even ostensibly positive stereotypes can be disadvantageous. A survey of Asian women in Coventry (Gray et al, 1993), for example, found that changes in the nature of work were leading managers increasingly to seek employees who were flexible, able to exercise initiative, and ready to carry responsibility for checking their own work and acquiring new skills. While employers were frequently ready to characterise Asian women workers as loyal, hardworking and uncomplaining, they also argued that these 'positive' qualities were no longer what was required by the demands of the modern workplace and labour market. Examples such as these dramatically reveal how easy it is for the routines of everyday working life to disadvantage minority ethnic groups even when there is no intention to discriminate. They also make it easy to hide intentional discrimination as the unplanned and accidental outcome of the market place.

Self-employment

It is a commonplace, confirmed by both the 1991 Census and the fourth PSI survey (Modood, 1997b), that self-employment is more common among minority ethnic groups than among the white population, although there are significant differences among minority ethnic groups. Among those classifying themselves into one of the 'Black' groups, self-employment is markedly less common than among the white population, while among those classified as 'Asian' it is considerably more common. Here again there are variations among Asian groups, Bangladeshis being less likely to be self-employed than other South Asians (Owen, 1993, pp 4-6; Modood, 1997b, pp 122-9). The pattern is similar for both male and female populations, although among African Asian women, levels of self-employment are similar to white women, and in all groups a larger proportion of men are self-employed. Labour Force Survey data also indicate that self-employment is generally concentrated into a restricted range of activities, with distribution, hotels, repairs and catering making up the largest areas of self-employment among all groups. Retail distribution is particularly prominent among the African Asian, Indian and Pakistani populations (Jones, 1993, pp 65-6).

These data appear to confirm a number of popular stereotypes: of unbusinesslike African-Caribbeans and of the thriving 'Asian' corner shop. In practice, several studies have drawn attention to the difficulties faced by entrepreneurs from minority ethnic groups (see, for example, Ward and Jenkins, 1984). In particular, there is evidence that minority ethnic businesses are often undercapitalised, recent research suggesting that African-Caribbean businesses have particular difficulties in accessing bank finance (Barrett, 1999). Other work has shown that minority ethnic businesses frequently operate on the margins of profitability and are dependent on a narrow, if relatively protected, ethnic market (Robinson, 1989, p 263).

Self-employment is often presented as a way for members of minority groups to escape the effects of discrimination in the labour market – an argument also hinted at in the discussion of the independent professions above. As Ram (1992) has argued, racism, indeed, is often a key factor in pushing minority groups into self-employment. However, Ram also argues that the effects of racism are not easy to transcend, and shows that many ethnic minority entrepreneurs find it difficult to escape the limits of an ethnically defined market in practice. One measure of this is that they frequently have to use white intermediaries or agents, and sometimes have deliberately to appoint white people to managerial posts, in order to develop appropriate contacts and establish credibility with customers.

In addition, Ram's analysis draws attention to the critical role played by the family as a resource in negotiating racism. This asset is not, however, without cost. Thus, family obligations may inhibit decisions that might otherwise be seen as economically rational. More critically, Ram suggests, such arrangements have specific implications for women. In particular, women are rarely defined as 'managers'. This role is assumed by men who constitute the external face of the firm. However, women play critical roles in the internal management of the enterprise, balancing conflicting demands and deploying human and financial resources. Typically, however, not only do these contributions go unacknowledged, but women are also usually simultaneously responsible for the domestic sphere. This point may be important to bear in mind in assessing the evidence of differential economic activity rates.

Household incomes and poverty

At the beginning of this chapter, it was argued that an understanding of employment was a key to understanding many other aspects of ethnic stratification. This is because labour market placement is central to the distribution of material resources and these in turn give access to a range of other resources and opportunities. To this end, we have thus far concentrated on patterns of labour market inclusion and exclusion and reviewed evidence about changing patterns of occupational mobility. We have also noted that there is at least some evidence that earnings may be beginning to reflect the upward mobility we have identified. Unfortunately, it turns out that matters are not that simple. In fact, there is not a straightforward relationship between occupational placement, earnings and the resources available to households.

The fourth PSI survey (Modood et al, 1997) attempted for the first time to produce an analysis of the *household* incomes of minority ethnic groups. This is important because the household is commonly used as the unit of analysis in discussions of living standards and economic well-being. We saw earlier that minority ethnic groups differed from one another and (with the exception of the African Asian and Chinese ethnic groups) from whites in *individual* earnings. It is a plausible assumption that individual earnings differences would be likely to feed through into household differences but the manner in which this takes place is not clear. Among relevant factors influencing outcomes will be relative household size, the number of wage earners and dependants and the availability of sources of income other than earnings. In this context, it is worth recalling that there are significant differences between groups in the size and structure of households and in family forms (Chapter Three of this volume; Berthoud, nd). These have particularly important implications for disposable resources and hence for the benefits accruing to employment. The analysis undertaken for the PSI reveals that the outcomes are complex and influenced by a range of factors. It also shows that, while some of the patterns revealed by analyses of employment continue to hold, there are other patterns that differ (Berthoud, 1997, pp 150-84; see also Berthoud, 1998).

The analysis is too complex to summarise adequately here. However, there are some matters of particular note. In particular, only Chinese households have incomes close to those of white households. Caribbean, Indian and African Asian households were all more likely than white households to experience poverty and less likely to have large family incomes. In the context of the evidence on upward occupational mobility reviewed earlier, we should note that, when incomes are taken into account, a somewhat less optimistic picture is revealed. When this is done, African Asians as well as Indians fare less well than those of Chinese descent, while Caribbeans are much better placed than Pakistanis and Bangladeshis (Berthoud, 1997, p 180). These data thus provide further reasons to be cautious when assessing the significance of occupational mobility and the relative labour market placement of groups.

It is also worth revisiting at this point the issue of economic activity. We saw earlier that economic activity rates, particularly for women, vary significantly from group to group. Data on patterns of employment appear to suggest that women from some ethnic groups have very low levels of economic activity. We should not too readily assume, however, that all of those omitted from the employment figures abstain from paid (as distinct from unpaid domestic) work. In the discussion of self-employment earlier, reference was made to hidden family labour – particularly of women. There is considerable evidence to suggest that official figures also seriously underestimate the volume of homeworking in the economy (Allen and Wolkowitz, 1987, especially ch 2; Felstead and Jewson, 1996, 1999). In its most exploitative forms, homeworking frequently preys upon women who, for childcare or other domestic reasons, are unable to engage in paid employment outside the home (Bisset and Huws, nd; Allen and Wolkowitz, 1987). There is also evidence that women in some minority ethnic groups are particularly likely, for cultural or other reasons, to be engaged in homeworking (Allen and Wolkowitz, 1987). To the extent that this is so, it alerts us to a largely hidden aspect of disadvantage. Key features of homeworking – particularly in textile and light assembly industries – often include very low rates of pay, and long and demanding hours of work (Bisset and Huws, nd; Felstead and Jewson, 1996, 1999). Thus, it may well be that, among those officially recorded as economically inactive, there are large numbers of women who are subject to particularly exploitative conditions of work with knock-on effects for household incomes.

One consequence of these features is that the effects of low incomes translate directly, in the case of the least well-placed groups (where several factors may converge) into significant levels of poverty. In this context, we should note in particular the prevalence of poverty (defined as incomes below half the national average) among Pakistani and Bangladeshi households. As Berthoud has put it:

Name any group whose poverty causes national concern – pensioners, disabled people, one-parent families, the unemployed – Pakistanis and Bangladeshis are poorer. (1997, p 180)

Conclusion

This chapter has attempted to track the changing terrain of labour market experiences of Britain's minority ethnic groups. It has noted the extent to which those experiences are characterised by considerable diversity as well as by both continuities and discontinuities over time. It has also noted the extent to which there may be cause for optimism about the trajectories of at least some groups (and on some analyses all groups). At the same time, it has identified a continuing ethnic penalty affecting all such groups to some degree; one that it is difficult to dissociate from continued discrimination. Finally, it has noted that, notwithstanding the pivotal position of the labour market in shaping overall life chances, the analysis of household incomes indicates that there is no straightforward, one-to-one, relationship between upward occupational mobility and household incomes. In particular, the circumstances of Pakistani and Bangladeshi families illustrate how a complex of factors can lead to multiple disadvantages that in turn have implications for other aspects of well-being. It is to some of these that this volume now turns.

Notes

[1] I am indebted to David Owen for these data.

[2] See also the discussion in Heath and McMahon (2000, especially pp 18-20).

[3] For a full discussion, see Modood (1997b, pp 112-17).

[4] Compare the discussion in Heath and McMahon (2000).

SIX

Patterns of and explanations for ethnic inequalities in health

James Y. Nazroo

Introduction

Since the early 1970s, ethnic differences in health have become an increasing focus of research in Britain. During this time, there have been extensive analyses of mortality data, using country of birth as a surrogate for ethnicity (for example, Marmot et al, 1984; Balarajan and Bulusu, 1990; Harding and Maxwell, 1997). There has also been a growing number of regional (for example, Pilgrim et al, 1993) and national surveys of ethnic differences in morbidity (for example, Rudat, 1994; Nazroo, 1997, 2001a; Johnson et al, 2000; Erens et al, 2001). This growing body of research reflects, at least in part, public policy concern with the health of, and quality of healthcare provided for, minority ethnic groups.

In theory, research should lead to policy developments that improve each of these aspects, but in practice this may not be the case. This is not only because research can be poorly disseminated, or because it may provide unpalatable messages to those concerned with public finance, but also because the research itself may contribute to the racialisation of health issues. The health disadvantage of minority ethnic groups is identified as somehow inherent to their ethnicity, a consequence of their cultural and genetic 'weaknesses', rather than a result of the disadvantages that they face as a result of the ways in which their ethnicity or 'race' is perceived by others.

Indeed, despite the extensive data-collection efforts and analyses cited earlier, the factors underlying ethnic differences in mortality and morbidity remain contested, and there continues to be debate around how far differences might be attributable to the disadvantaged social circumstances in which minority ethnic people are more likely to live. For example, as long ago as 1845, Engels attributed the poor health of Irish people living in England to the poor social circumstances in which the majority of the Irish population lived (Engels, 1987). On the other hand, some claim that socioeconomic inequalities make a minimal contribution – or else none at all – to ethnic inequalities in health (Wild and McKeigue, 1997). Others suggest that, even if they do contribute, the cultural and genetic elements of ethnicity must also play a role (Smaje, 1996).

Given the growing sophistication of this field, it is worrying that crude explanations based on cultural stereotypes and claims of genetic difference persist (see, for example, Soni Raleigh and Balarajan, 1992; Gupta et al, 1995; Stewart et al, 1999). And all this despite a lack of concrete evidence and more than 100 years of research exposing the limitations of the assumptions underlying such explanations (for example, Bhopal, 1997).

This chapter exposes some of the assumptions that have underpinned much of the research and policy debate in relation to ethnic differences in health, and illustrates how far such differences are likely to be a consequence of the social inequalities faced by minority ethnic people in Britain. First, data are presented that show how ethnic inequalities in health in Britain are patterned. Particular attention is paid to the importance of careful ethnic categorisation for an accurate description. The chapter then explores various explanations for ethnic inequalities in health, and exposes how some are rooted in crude notions of cultural and genetic difference. Next, the chapter demonstrates how socioeconomic inequalities are too readily dismissed as a potential explanation for ethnic inequalities in health and, in fact, may be a crucial explanation. Finally, the chapter shows how experiences of racial harassment and discrimination might also lead to an increased risk of poor health.

The ethnic patterning of health

What follows is brief description of ethnic variations in health, primarily relying on morbidity data from the Policy Studies Institute Fourth National Survey of Ethnic Minorities (FNS) (Nazroo, 1997, 2001a) and the 1999 Health Survey for England (HSE) (Erens et al, 2001). In addition to these sources are analyses of migrant mortality data conducted by ONS for the period 1991-93 (Harding and Maxwell, 1997; Maxwell and Harding, 1998).

Figure 6.1, drawn from the HSE, provides an overview of ethnic inequalities in health. It shows differences in a broad indicator of morbidity, self-reported general health, across ethnic groups for adults and children aged two or older. It charts the odds ratio and 95% confidence intervals, in comparison with a white English group, for reporting health as fair or bad, rather than good. Immediately obvious is the heterogeneity in experience across ethnic groups. Most notable is the wide variation for the three South Asian groups – Indian, Pakistani and Bangladeshi – who are typically treated as one and the same ethnic group (for example, McKeigue et al, 1988; Gupta et al, 1995).

Tables 6.1 and 6.2 provide more detail, showing mortality and morbidity differences for some more specific outcomes. Table 6.1 summarises findings from the most recent analysis of immigrant mortality around the 1991 Census, showing age standardised mortality ratios (SMRs) by country of birth for all causes and four specific causes of death (chosen for illustrative purposes). Table 6.2 provides a summary of data on morbidity for the adult population, and is drawn from the FNS. It shows the relative risk for minority ethnic people compared with white people to report fair or poor health and indicators of

Figure 6.1: Ethnic differences in reported fair or bad general health in Britain

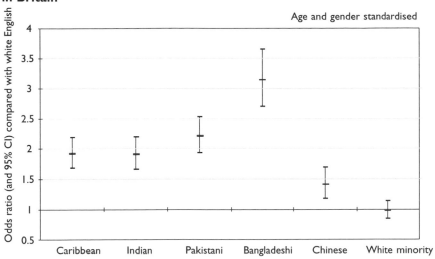

CI = confidence intervals
Source: Health Survey for England (1999)

four specific conditions (a combination of responses to questions on previously diagnosed conditions and symptoms).

Some general interpretations can be taken from Figure 6.1 and Tables 6.1 and 6.2. First, minority ethnic groups are not uniformly at greater risk of mortality or poor health. For example, both the mortality data and the FNS morbidity data suggest that Indian people have reasonably good overall health. Second, for some outcomes minority ethnic groups appear to be significantly better off than the ethnic majority (for example, respiratory symptoms/disease and lung cancer). Third, particular ethnic groups appear to be disadvantaged by different diseases. For example, Caribbean people have high rates of stroke/ hypertension and South Asian people have high rates of coronary heart disease/ severe chest pain. Fourth, the morbidity data reveal great heterogeneity in experience among the South Asian groups, with Indian people reporting better health than Pakistani or Bangladeshi people, and levels of health that are on a par with those of the white majority.

Although there are similarities in the data presented in the two tables, there are also some inconsistencies. For example, Caribbean people have a low all-cause standardised mortality ratio (SMR), but high relative risk of reporting fair or poor general health. Those born in India have an elevated SMR for coronary heart disease, while their relative risk for a diagnosis or reporting symptoms of heart disease is lower than that for white people. South Asian people have a high SMR from stroke but a lower relative risk of reporting hypertension. These inconsistencies could be a consequence of a number of factors, including:

Table 6.1: Standardised mortality ratio by country of birth for those aged 20-64, England and Wales (1991-93)

	All causes		Coronary heart disease		Stroke		Respiratory disease		Lung cancer	
	M	W	M	W	M	W	M	W	M	W
Caribbean	89[a]	104	60[a]	100	169[a]	178[a]	80[a]	75	59[a]	32[a]
Indian subcontinent	107[a]	99	150[a]	175[a]	163[a]	132[a]	90	94	48[a]	34[a]
India	106[a]	–	140[a]	–	140[a]	–	93	–	43[a]	–
Pakistan	102	–	163[a]	–	148[a]	–	82	–	45[a]	–
Bangladesh	137[a]	–	184[a]	–	324[a]	–	104	–	92	–
East Africa	123[a]	127[a]	160[a]	130	113	110	154[a]	195[a]	35[a]	110
West/ South Africa	126[a]	142[a]	83	69	315[a]	215[a]	138	101	71	69
Ireland	135[a]	115[a]	121[a]	129[a]	130[a]	118[a]	162[a]	134[a]	157[a]	143[a]

M = men; w = women

[a] $p < 0.05$

Source: Harding and Maxwell (1997), Maxwell and Harding (1998)

Table 6.2: Age- and gender-standardised relative risk, all ages, England and Wales (1993-94)

	Fair or poor health	Diagnosed heart disease	Heart disease or severe chest pain	Hypertension	Diabetes	Respiratory symptoms
Caribbean	1.29[a]	0.88	0.96	1.47[a]	3.12[a]	0.87
All South Asian	1.19[a]	1.00	1.24[a]	0.75[a]	3.65[a]	0.59[a]
Indian	1.03	0.79	0.93	0.66[a]	2.77[a]	0.55[a]
Pakistani or Bangladeshi	1.48[a]	1.43[a]	1.83[a]	0.91	5.24[a]	0.67[a]
Chinese	0.96	0.71	0.56	0.42[a]	1.77	0.43[a]

[a] $p < 0.05$

Source: Nazroo (1997)

- the data cover different groups (the mortality data are restricted to those born outside the UK, while the morbidity data cover all minority ethnic people, but only those aged 16+);
- the morbidity data measure prevalence while the mortality data measure a combination of incidence and survival (in the UK, there is of course some out-migration which will particularly bias the mortality statistics);
- there may be important cohort effects present;
- there may be data inaccuracies both in the reporting of symptoms or diagnosis (perhaps because of cultural differences in the experience and reporting of symptoms or differences in opportunities for diagnosis) and in the recording of cause of death, as there appear to be for occupational class and gender (Battle et al, 1987; Bloor et al, 1989).

All of this points to a need for a critical questioning of data:

- how comprehensive is the coverage of the data (nationally representative, covering both immigrants and British born minority ethnic people)?
- how valid and reliable are the health measures included?
- perhaps most important of all, how adequate is the assignment of ethnicity to individuals in the data? And does it reflect the heterogeneity of ethnic groups? Is observer-assigned ethnicity used instead of self-reported ethnicity, and are surrogates such as country of birth used instead of ethnic origin?

Genetic and cultural explanations for ethnic differences in health

While some of the mainstream research and policy criticisms of essentialised notions of 'race' and culture appear to have been adopted by research on ethnicity and health, this often happens in a presentational rather than an analytical way. Within British studies, 'race' is never explicitly measured and 'ethnicity' is clearly the term favoured for describing health differences across minority groups. However, the nature of quantitative health (epidemiological) research, with a need for easily used and repeatable measures, often results in the poor measurement of ethnic categories. The concepts of ethnicity and race are often merged (despite the exclusive use of the term ethnicity) and the dynamic and contextual nature of ethnicity are ignored. So, the term 'ethnic' is frequently used to refer to genetic and cultural features that are undesirable (from a health perspective) and inherent to the minority groups under investigation.

Before going on to explore why research on ethnicity and health tends to be reduced to genetic and cultural explanations, and how this can be avoided, it is worth illustrating this point with two examples. The first concerns the well-publicised greater risk for 'South Asians' in Britain of coronary heart disease. An editorial in the *British Medical Journal* (Gupta et al, 1995) used research findings to attribute this problem to a combination of genetic (race) and cultural (ethnicity) factors that are apparently associated with being 'South Asian'. Concerning genetics, the suggestion was that 'South Asians' have a shared evolutionary history that involved adaptation "to survive under conditions of periodic famine and low energy intake" (p 1035). This resulted in the development of 'insulin resistance syndrome', which apparently underlies 'South Asians" greater risk of coronary heart disease. From this perspective 'South Asians' can be viewed as a genetically distinct group with a unique evolutionary history – that is, a race. In terms of cultural factors, the use of ghee in cooking, a lack of physical exercise and a reluctance to use health services were all mentioned[1].

It is important to note how the policy recommendations flowing from such an approach underline the extent to which the issue has become racialised. The authors of the editorial recommend that 'community leaders' and 'survivors' of heart attacks should spread the message among their communities and that 'South Asians' should be encouraged to undertake healthier lifestyles (Gupta et al, 1995). Apparently, the problem of high rates of coronary heart disease is viewed as something inherent to being 'South Asian' – nothing to do with the context of the lives of 'South Asians' – and as only solvable if 'South Asians' are encouraged to modify their behaviours to address their genetic and cultural weaknesses.

The second example involves the high mortality rates from suicide among young women living in Britain who were born on the Indian subcontinent. Attempts to explain this have focused on cultural explanations, particularly on a notion of culture conflict, where the young woman is apparently in disagreement with her parents' (or husband's) traditional or religious expectations. For example, despite an almost complete lack of evidence, Soni Raleigh and Balarajan state:

> Most immigrant Asian communities have maintained their cultural identity and traditions even after generations of overseas residence. This tradition incorporates a premium on academic and economic success, a stigma attached to failure, the overriding authority of elders (especially parents and in-laws) and expected unquestioning compliance from younger family members.... These pressures are intensified in young Indian women, given their rigidly defined roles in Indian society. Submission and deference to males and elders, arranged marriages, the financial pressures imposed by dowries, and ensuing marital and family conflicts have been cited as contributory factors to suicide and attempted suicide in young Indian women in several of the studies reviewed here. (Soni Raleigh and Balarajan, 1992, p 367)

Again, such research has led to the racialisation of the issue. The problem is located within a relatively permanent and pathological culture, and one that needs to adopt the 'freedoms' allowed to young white women.

Both examples provide us with notions of groups that are (from a health point of view) genetically and culturally inferior to the white population.

Central to reaching such conclusions is the combination of the belief that comparative epidemiology can provide clues to aetiology, the assumption that ethnicity is a useful and easy tool for demarcating groups to provide the basis for comparison, and the crudeness with which ethnicity is measured in such work. The crudeness with which ethnicity is assessed in nearly all of this work allows the status of ethnicity as an explanatory variable to be assumed. The view of ethnicity as a *natural* division between social groups allows the *description* of ethnic variations in health to become their *explanation* (Sheldon and Parker, 1992; Ahmad, 1996). Consequently, explanations are based on cultural stereotypes or suppositions about genetic differences, rather than attempting directly to assess the nature and importance of such factors. Here it is worth emphasising the different status of explanations used for minority ethnic groups compared with the ethnic majority. While a lack of interest in exercise, or restrictive family practices, are a consequence of a pathological (minority) culture, high rates of smoking are not viewed as a problem arising from white ethnicity that should be ameliorated by a modification of white culture(s).

In fact, a more sensitive measurement of ethnicity can lead to quite different conclusions. For example, while Table 6.2 shows that, although South Asian people as a group had a greater risk of indicators of heart disease than white people, once the group was broken down into constituent parts this only applied to Pakistani and Bangladeshi people. Indian people had the same rate as white people (see Nazroo, 2001b, for a more detailed analysis of this). This does not mean that cultural or genetic factors are of no use in explaining poor health. Rather, cultural practices and genetic differences need to be directly assessed, rather than assumed, and the contexts in which they operate and their association with health outcomes measured. Also, other explanatory factors have to be considered when exploring the relationship between ethnicity and health, in particular those related to socioeconomic position.

Socioeconomic position and ethnic inequalities in health

Given the pattern of socioeconomic deprivation faced by some minority ethnic groups in Britain and the clearly established relationship between socioeconomic factors and health (Townsend and Davidson, 1982), it would be expected that minority ethnic people generally have poorer health as a result of their poorer class position. However, in Britain class has disappeared from investigations into the relationship between ethnicity and health, with one or two notable exceptions (Ahmad et al, 1989; Fenton et al, 1995; Smaje, 1995; Nazroo, 1997, 1998, 2001a). Instead, work in this field has largely followed a trend set by the now classic work of Marmot et al (1984). Their findings, based on an analysis of mortality rates by country of birth, indicated that class and (as a consequence) material explanations were unrelated to mortality rates for most immigrant groups. In addition, they made no contribution to the higher mortality rates found among those who had migrated to Britain. Indeed, for one group – those born in the 'Caribbean Commonwealth' – the relationship between class and overall mortality rates was the opposite of that for the general population. Marmot et al concluded:

> (a) that differences in social class distribution are not the explanation of the overall different mortality of migrants; and (b) the relation of social class (as usually defined) to mortality is different among immigrant groups from the England and Wales pattern. (Marmot et al, 1984, p 21)

Rather than puzzling over why such an important explanation for inequalities in health among the general population did not apply to minority ethnic groups, many researchers have simply accepted that different sets of explanations for poor health applied to ethnic minority and majority populations and, of course, that, for the minority population, explanations were related to cultural and genetic differences. There are, in fact, a number of reasons why the relationship between class and mortality rates might have been suppressed in these data. Most important is that Marmot et al used 'occupation' as recorded on death certificates to define social class. There is a well-recognised practice of relatives inflating the occupational status of the deceased person on the death certificate by declaring the most prestigious occupation held by him or her (Townsend and Davidson, 1982). It is likely, then, that this practice means that Marmot et al's recording technique fails to capture the downward social mobility of members of minority ethnic groups on migration to Britain (a process that both Smith, 1977, and Heath and Ridge, 1983, have documented). So, the occupation recorded on the death certificates of migrants may well be an inaccurate reflection of their experience in Britain prior to death. In addition, given the socioeconomic profile of minority ethnic groups in Britain, this inflation of occupational status would only need to happen in relatively few cases for the figures representing the small population in higher classes to be distorted upwards.

More recent data have challenged the conclusions reached by Marmot et al (1984). Figure 6.2 shows rates of reporting fair or poor health for three minority ethnic groups (in order to achieve large enough sample sizes, the Pakistani and Bangladeshi groups have been combined) and a comparative white sample using data from the FNS (Nazroo, 1997). Each of the groups is stratified by the occupational class of the head of the household, with a simple distinction drawn between manual and non-manual households, and a third group – those where there was no full-time worker in the household – also included. It shows a clear relationship between reported general health and socioeconomic position for each ethnic group. Important here is the suggestion that it is misleading, for example, to consider Caribbean people as uniformly disadvantaged in terms of their health. Those in better socioeconomic positions have better health; there is nothing inevitable, or inherent, in the link between being Caribbean, Bangladeshi and so on, and a greater risk of mortality and morbidity. However, the figure also raises the possibility that socioeconomic effects do not explain ethnic inequalities in health. Within each class group,

Figure 6.2: Reported fair, poor, or very poor health (by ethnic group and class)

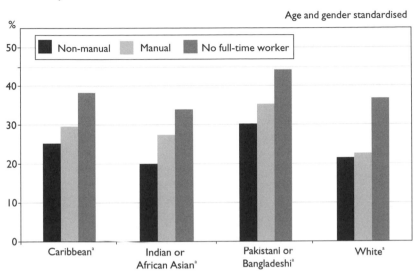

Age and gender standardised

ᵃ p <0.001

those in the Pakistani or Bangladeshi category were more likely than those in the white category to report fair or poor health. This might suggest that socioeconomic factors do not contribute to ethnic inequalities in health, even if health is patterned along socioeconomic lines within ethnic groups.

Similar findings were found in the most recent analysis of immigrant mortality data, conducted around the 1991 Census. This showed that socioeconomic differentials might be an important explanation of inequalities in mortality rates *within* minority ethnic groups, but still suggested that differences *between* ethnic groups remain unexplained by class effects, leading its authors to conclude that:

> ... social class is not an adequate explanation for the patterns of excess mortality observed [among migrant groups]. (Harding and Maxwell, 1997, p 120)

Given such findings, it might be tempting to believe that the differences between groups must be a consequence of 'obvious' genetic and cultural factors. However, it is important to recognise that important shortcomings remain in the statistics used. Most important is that the attempt to control for socioeconomic factors with an indicator such as occupational class ignores how crude this measure is and how it may apply differently to different ethnic groups. In fact, there has been an increasing recognition of the limitations of traditional class groupings, which are far from internally homogeneous. A number of studies have drawn attention to variations in income levels and death rates among occupations that comprise particular occupational classes (for example, Davey Smith et al,

1990). And within an occupational group, minority ethnic people may be more likely to be found in lower or less prestigious occupational grades, to have poorer job security, to endure more stressful working conditions and to be more likely to work unsocial hours.

So, the process of standardising for socioeconomic position when making comparisons across groups, particularly ethnic groups, is not as straightforward as it might at first sight seem. As Kaufman et al (1997, 1998) point out, the process of standardisation is effectively an attempt to deal with the non-random nature of samples used in cross-sectional population studies – controlling for all relevant 'extraneous' explanatory factors introduces the *appearance* of randomisation. However, attempting to introduce randomisation into cross-sectional studies by adding 'controls' has a number of problems, as summarised by Kaufman et al:

> When considering socioeconomic exposures and making comparisons between racial/ethnic groups ... the material, behavioral, and psychological circumstances of diverse socioeconomic and racial/ethnic groups are distinct on so many dimensions that no realistic adjustment can plausibly simulate randomization. (Kaufman et al, 1998, p 147)

Indeed, evidence from the FNS (Nazroo, 1997) illustrates this point clearly. The first part of Table 6.3 shows the mean equivalised household income for individuals within particular classes by ethnic group. Each ethnic group shows the expected income gradient by occupational class. However, when comparisons are drawn across ethnic groups, the table shows that, within each occupational class, Caribbean and Indian or African Asian people appear to

Table 6.3: Ethnic variations in socioeconomic position within socioeconomic bands

	White	Indian or African Asian	Pakistani or Bangladeshi	Caribbean
Mean income by Registrar General's class pounds[a]				
I/II	250	210	125	210
IIINM	185	135	95	145
IIIM	160	120	70	145
IV/V	130	110	65	120
Median duration of unemployment for those currently unemployed (months)	7	12	24	21

Notes: [a] Based on bands of equivalised household income. The mean point of each band is used to make this calculation, which is rounded to the nearest 5.

NM = non-manual; M = manual.

Source: Nazroo (1997)

have similar locations, while white people were better off than them and Pakistani or Bangladeshi people worse off than them. Indeed, comparing the white and Pakistani or Bangladeshi groups shows that, within each occupational class band, those in the Pakistani or Bangladeshi group had (on average) half the white income, and Class I or II Pakistani or Bangladeshi people had an equivalent average income to Class IV or V white people. This suggests that standardising for Registrar General's class is a far from adequate method of dealing with socioeconomic effects for comparisons across ethnic groups, even if this indicator does reflect socioeconomic differences within ethnic groups. The second part of the table shows the median length of unemployment for those who were currently unemployed at interview. It again shows diverse patterns across ethnic groups, with those in the white and Indian or African Asian groups having been unemployed for a considerably shorter period than those in the Caribbean and Pakistani or Bangladeshi groups. Here it is worth noting that Bartley et al (1996) clearly showed that length of unemployment, rather than unemployment per se, was an important determinant of health.

The overall conclusion, then, is that using single or crude indicators of socioeconomic position is of little use for 'controlling out' the impact of socioeconomic position when attempting to reveal the extent of a 'non-socioeconomic' ethnic/race effect. Within any given level of a particular socioeconomic indicator, the social circumstances of minority ethnic people in Britain are less favourable than those of white people. Therefore, while the presentation of 'standardised' data allows the reader to assume that all

Figure 6.3: Relative risk of fair, poor, or very poor health standardised for socioeconomic factors: Pakistani or Bangladeshi group compared with white groups

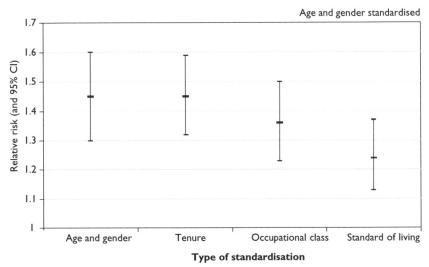

CI = confidence intervals

that is left is an 'ethnic/race' effect – be that cultural or genetic. The problems with such data, outlined by Kaufman et al (1997, 1998) and illustrated by Table 6.3, suggest that very little, if anything, is really being standardised for.

Nevertheless, when such difficulties are considered carefully, there are some benefits in attempting to control for socioeconomic effects. In particular, if controlling for socioeconomic effects alters the pattern of ethnic inequalities in health, despite the limitations of the indicators used, we can conclude that at least some of the differences we have uncovered are a result of a socioeconomic effect. This possibility is supported by Figure 6.3, which uses data from the FNS to show changes in the relative risk of reporting fair or poor health for the Pakistani or Bangladeshi group compared with white people once the data had been standardised for a variety of socioeconomic factors. A comparison of the first bar with the second and third shows that standardising for occupational class and tenure, standard socioeconomic variables in British epidemiological studies, makes no difference. However, taking account of an indicator of 'standard of living' – a more direct reflection of the economic circumstances of respondents (see Nazroo, 1997, 2001a, for full details) – leads to a large reduction in the relative risk (compare the first and last bars). Although this indicator is not perfect for taking account of ethnic differences in socioeconomic status (Nazroo, 1997, Table 5.4), such a finding suggests that socioeconomic differences, in fact, make a large and key contribution to ethnic inequalities in health.

Figure 6.4: Reduction in (ln) odds ratio of reporting fair or bad health compared with white English after adjusting for socioeconomic effects

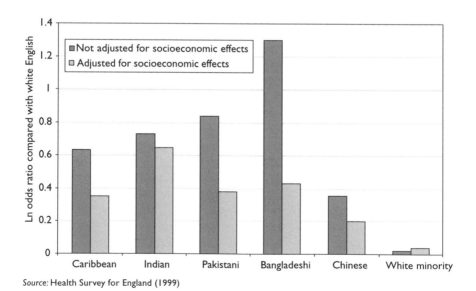

Source: Health Survey for England (1999)

This impression is strengthened when the process is repeated across ethnic groups and across outcomes. Figure 6.4 uses data from the HSE to explore the impact of socioeconomic factors on ethnic differences in reporting fair or bad general health across a range of ethnic groups. Once adjustments had been made simultaneously for a variety of socioeconomic indicators (income, housing tenure, economic activity), there is a clear and large reduction in odds ratio for most minority ethnic groups (the natural logarithm of the odds ratio in comparison with white English people is used, to give an accurate visual impression of the size of change in odds). Exceptions are the white minority group (which has an odds close to 1) and the Indian group.

Figure 6.5 uses data from the FNS to explore the impact of socioeconomic factors across three broad minority ethnic groups and six outcomes (Nazroo,

Figure 6.5: Reduction in (ln) relative risk of ill health compared with white people after controlling for standard of living

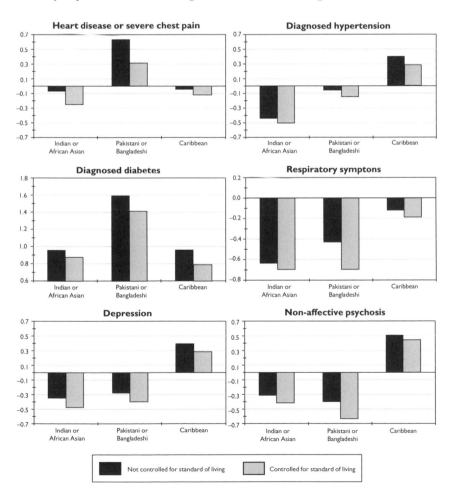

2001a). It shows the natural logarithm of the relative risk statistic to compare how the risk of ill health across the six health dimensions changes for minority ethnic respondents compared with white respondents (once socioeconomic position is partially adjusted for using the standard of living indicator). In Figure 6.5, a risk equivalent to that for white people is represented by the X-axis (the value 0), and a figure above this represents a greater risk, while a figure below this a smaller risk. In all cases, the risk for each minority ethnic group compared with white people is reduced once the socioeconomic control has been applied.

Figures 6.3–6.5 have suggested that differences in socioeconomic position make a key contribution to ethnic inequalities in health, particularly when we take seriously the cautions on the difficulties with making effective adjustments for socioeconomic position. It is also worth emphasising that the analyses shown here simply reflect current socioeconomic position. Data on the life course and on other forms of social disadvantage were not included and are almost universally not available in existing studies of ethnic inequalities in health. Nevertheless, it is worth considering the impact of other forms of social disadvantage on risk of poor health, in particular, in the case of ethnic inequalities in health, experiences of racism.

Impact of experiences of racial harassment and discrimination on health

Experiences and awareness of racism appear to be central to the lives of minority ethnic people. Qualitative investigations of experience of racial harassment and discrimination have found that, for many people, experiences of interpersonal racism are a part of everyday life, that the way they lead their lives is constrained by fear of racial harassment, and that being made to feel different is routine and expected (Virdee, 1995; Chalal and Julienne, 1999). Findings from the FNS suggested widespread experiences of racial harassment and discrimination among minority ethnic people in Britain:

- more than one in eight respondents reported having experienced at least one incident of harassment over the preceding year (Virdee, 1997);
- there was a widespread belief among minority ethnic respondents that employers discriminated against minority ethnic applicants for jobs, and widespread experience of such discrimination (Modood, 1997b);
- when white people were asked about their opinions, one in five said that they were racially prejudiced against Caribbean people and one in four said they were racially prejudiced against Asian people (Virdee, 1997).

In the few studies that have been conducted, experiences of racial harassment and discrimination appear to be related to health. Studies in the US have shown a relationship between self-reported experiences of racial harassment and a range of health outcomes, including hypertension, psychological distress, poorer self-rated health and days spent unwell in bed. The studies also found that differences in rates of hypertension between black and white respondents were substantially reduced by taking into account reported experiences of, and responses to, racial harassment (James et al, 1987; Krieger et al, 1993; Krieger and Sidney, 1996). In Britain, analyses of the FNS also suggested a relationship between experiences of racial harassment, perceptions of racial discrimination and a range of health outcomes across ethnic groups (Karlsen and Nazroo, 2002a). Table 6.4, drawn from these analyses, shows that reporting experiences of racial harassment and the perception that employers discriminate against minority ethnic people are independently related to likelihood of reporting fair or poor health, and that this relationship is independent of socioeconomic effects. It may be that this represents three dimensions of social and economic inequality operating simultaneously:

*   economic disadvantage (as measured by occupational class);
*   a sense of being a member of a devalued, low-status group (British employers discriminate);
*   the personal insult and stress of being a victim of racial harassment.

Conclusion

Despite the breadth of data on ethnic inequalities in health in Britain, there remain ongoing problems with the quality of available data. Studies often do not contain sufficiently detailed information on the ethnicity of respondents

Table 6.4: Racial harassment, racial discrimination and risk of fair or poor health

| | All ethnic minority groups | |
	Odds ratio[a]	95% confidence intervals
Experience of racial harassment		
No attack	1.00	–
Verbal abuse	1.54	1.07-2.21
Physical attack	2.07	1.14-3.76
Perception of discrimination		
Fewer than half of employers discriminate	1.00	–
Most employers discriminate	1.39	1.10-1.76
Occupational class		
Non-manual	1.00	–
Manual	1.44	1.07-1.94
No full-time worker in the household	2.42	1.82-3.22

[a] Adjusted for gender and age.

Source: Karlsen and Nazroo (2002a)

to reflect heterogeneity across ethnic groups and heterogeneity within broadly defined ethnic groups. Socioeconomic data are either not collected at all, or are collected at very crude levels that are plainly inadequate for drawing comparisons across ethnic groups. Those socioeconomic data that are collected invariably reflect current position, rather than risks across the life course. And they do not include other dimensions of social inequality, such as experiences of racial harassment and discrimination.

Nevertheless, a large body of convincing evidence now supports the possibility that ethnic inequalities in health are largely a consequence of socioeconomic differentials. This applies across a range of minority ethnic groups and a range of outcomes. Furthermore, there is a growing body of evidence suggesting that experiences of racial harassment and discrimination, and perceptions of living in a discriminatory society, contribute to ethnic inequalities in health. Also, there are other dimensions of social inequality faced by minority ethnic groups that might lead to health inequalities. For example, the specific geographical locations of minority ethnic people might be an important source of social disadvantage. In addition, a growing body of evidence shows the importance of geographical inequalities and how these might operate to result in inequalities in health (Macintyre et al, 1993; Sloggett and Joshi, 1994). It is clear that minority ethnic people are more likely to be found in the most 'unhealthy' areas (Karlsen and Nazroo, 2002b).

The evidence of inequalities in access to health services also continues to grow. Although a number of studies have shown that minority ethnic people are at least as likely as white people to consult with their GP (Rudat, 1994; Nazroo, 1997; Erens et al, 2001), they are less likely to leave the surgery with a follow-up appointment (Gilliam et al, 1989), or to receive follow-up services such as a district nurse (Badger et al, 1989). More detailed enquiries have suggested that South Asian people with coronary heart disease wait longer for referral to specialist care than white people (Shaukat et al, 1993) despite appearing to be more likely to seek immediate care (Ben-Shlomo et al, 1996). None of these studies has been able to explore reasons for these possible differences in quality of care. However, it has been shown that minority ethnic people are more likely than white people to:

- find physical access to their GP difficult;
- have longer waiting times in the surgery;
- feel that the time their GP had spent with them was inadequate;
- to be unhappy with the outcome of the consultation (Rudat 1994).

Part of this might be related to communication problems. In terms of language, a significant number of South Asian (particularly Bangladeshi women) and Chinese people find it difficult to communicate with their GP (Nazroo, 1997). And many minority ethnic women prefer to consult with female doctors, and, in order to overcome communication difficulties, female doctors with the same minority ethnic background as themselves (Nazroo, 1997).

However, the findings that suggest the importance of social and economic disadvantage to ethnic inequalities in health need to be placed within a wider explanatory framework. Here it is important to consider the centrality of racism to any attempt to explain ethnic inequalities in health. Not only are personal experiences of racism and harassment likely to impact on health, but racism as a social force will play a central role in structuring the social and economic disadvantage faced by minority ethnic groups. The socioeconomic differences between ethnic groups should not be considered as somehow autonomous. The process of postwar immigration of minority ethnic people to Britain and the socioeconomic disadvantage faced by minority ethnic immigrants subsequently was, and continues to be, structured by racism that has its roots in colonial history (Gilroy, 1987; Miles, 1989). Indeed, there is a need to recognise the overriding importance of national and historical context on the 'making' of ethnic groups, how this is related to economic processes and inequities in this, and how this influences the lives of minority ethnic and migrant populations. It is entirely possible that racism is involved at a fundamental level in the structuring of economic, social and health opportunities for minority ethnic people.

Note

[1] Ghee is not, however, used by all of the ethnic groups that comprise 'South Asians'. Furthermore, evidence suggests that 'South Asians' do understand the importance of exercise (Beishon and Nazroo, 1997) and do use medical services (Rudat, 1994; Nazroo, 1997; Erens et al, 2001).

SEVEN

Housing black and minority ethnic communities: diversity and constraint

Malcolm Harrison

Introduction

The housing experiences of minority ethnic households arc very varied, and negative stereotypes of segregation into so-called 'ghetto' life tell us little about the meanings or shifting characteristics of home and community. Diverse trajectories have become more visible in recent years between and across specific minority ethnic groups, and there are many housing success stories. Yet there is also a continuity of shared disadvantages for communities, affecting opportunities, resources and housing choice. Furthermore, patterns associated with socioeconomic differentiation, gender and disability may cross-cut or reinforce those associated with ethnicity.

This chapter draws on a review commissioned in 2001 by the then Department for Transport, Local Government and the Regions, designed to appraise the evidence base in the field of housing for black and minority ethnic households in England (Harrison with Phillips, 2003). In reviewing the 'state of the art' for housing research, we noted the richness and extensiveness of existing empirical materials, but also many gaps in knowledge. Analysis by policy makers and scholars has often relied on anecdotal or very localised findings. This is partly because housing conditions and decisions are so complex and particular, and large-scale surveys can rarely cater for the detail. Not only do dwellings vary in age, affordability, type and tenure, they are the focus for activities by a wide range of organisations in private and non-profit spheres, with local and regional variations in markets, costs and capital values. The housing options open to people from a specific minority ethnic group may differ from place to place, reflecting factors such as house prices or the availability of social rented dwellings, as well as labour market opportunities. Thus, differences in location can connect to differing patterns in the housing circumstances of specific minority ethnic groups. For instance, Howes and Mullins (1999) have noted that, while Bangladeshi people in London were found to be particularly likely to be council housing tenants (58%), this appeared much less the case for those living elsewhere in Britain (only 15% of whom were apparently local authority tenants). At the same time, housing supply complications may be paralleled by variations in household circumstances and strategies linked to gender, community or settlement histories, religious or kinship affiliations, age, disability, health, or incomes. Thus, the housing scene is a highly complicated mosaic of varying conditions, resources and opportunities.

Systematic data are scarce on several fronts. Little is known about recent trends in the performance of private landlords, lettings agents, or financial services in responding to diverse communities and needs. The lack of information about the behaviour of market intermediaries, lenders and financial services is problematic, although there are insights from localised qualitative research. Bowes et al (1997a), for example, have indicated reluctance of building societies to fund mortgages for Pakistani families in Glasgow, although acknowledging that societies have not generally displayed "the same anti-Asian sentiments as estate agents" (1997a, p 81). Very recently, Phillips has surveyed estate agents in Leeds, suggesting that discriminatory practices may be persisting (see Harrison with Phillips, 2003, p 46). Other topics where information is limited concern housing quality and the costs experienced by households (which ideally would be linked up with data on incomes, affordability and financial services, including access to insurance). In addition, we have few data on the housing capital possessed by specific minorities, and the terms on which assets are acquired or held. As regards households, not enough is known on housing in relation to chronic illness and disability, gender, the implications of housing conditions for children, and the circumstances of 'newer' or 'less visible' minority and migrant groups. Furthermore, only a small number of substantial studies have begun to consider the complexities of housing 'pathways' and trajectories for minority ethnic households (although see Bowes et al, 1997a, 1997b, 1998; Harrison with Phillips, 2003). It remains difficult to link housing experiences with what is happening in education, health or employment. For example, we do not know whether, or how far, educational successes within households are matched by improved housing quality, or are gained at the expense of sacrificing the latter. We cannot say with certainty whether housing advance is subject to more persistent obstacles than those experienced in other fields.

Despite these deficiencies, there is plenty of material indicating ongoing disadvantage. Circumstances are best described by the term 'difference within difference', which captures the sense that the UK's society is still characterised by a major patterning of outcomes in which the 'white/black minority ethnic' divide remains significant, even though differentiation at the level of household or minority group experiences is great (for this concept in relation to disability, ethnicity and gender, see Harrison with Davis, 2001). In a situation of 'difference within difference', it remains appropriate to refer to *ethnic penalties*, especially insofar as constraints continue to affect housing and area choice. Although deploying the word 'ethnic' in this context may not capture fully what is happening, the terminology nonetheless has been used effectively by writers to denote situations whereby members of non-white groups (regardless of qualifications and positions in jobs hierarchies) tend to suffer a disadvantage that leads them to fare less well than apparently comparable white people (Karn, 1997, pp 266-7, 275-81; Modood et al, 1997, pp 144-5). Noting a continuity and commonality of disadvantage does not mean setting aside the vitality of specific cultures, the impact of collective actions in securing changes, or the capacity of individual households to make progress. Rather, it acknowledges that barriers persist, alongside the potential for constructive change and the rich cultural resources that some groups draw upon.

Difference within difference: diversity but persisting barriers

There are marked differences between various minority ethnic communities in terms of households, tenure patterns, dwelling types, settlement geographies, and density of occupation (see Ratcliffe, 1997). Changing household sizes and structures and population age structures are important. Different groups have differing population growth rates and potential for new household formation, with implications for patterns of future local housing needs (Phillips, 1996). There may be particular difficulties in meeting those needs where growth occurs in communities with low incomes located in 'tight' housing markets where affordable housing is overcrowded and in short supply. Although we tend to associate housing market pressures with the South East of England, some communities in northern cities live in poor-quality dwellings and experience a combination of problems of overcrowding, poor health, low incomes and limitations on housing choice and safe outward movement (discussed later in this chapter).

As far as tenure is concerned, recent figures suggest that a fifth of Indian heads of household in England own their house outright, compared with only one in 20 of those heads of households from the Black and Bangladeshi groups. A further 55% of Indian households apparently own with a mortgage. While there may be patterns of underrepresentation in council housing for Asian groups as a whole, it is necessary to disaggregate to gain a proper picture. In England, the Black and Bangladeshi groups overall are by far the most likely among the black minority ethnic groups to be renting from the social rented housing sectors (see Matheson and Pullinger, 1999, p 170; compare Ratcliffe, 1997, pp 133-8). Data for London suggest that the total number of black minority ethnic social renting tenants there increased from around 90,000 in the late 1970s to 244,000 in the mid-1990s, despite an overall decline in numbers of such tenancies (Housing Corporation London, 1999, p 16). Nationally, housing associations are significant for some minority ethnic households, while the role played by social renting for female-headed households is, of course, important (just as it is among white households), not least because of the problems single parents face in other tenures.

Along with differences between minority ethnic groups, there are also variable experiences *within* minority categories according to generation, gender, household type and socioeconomic status. Impairment and chronic illness are likely to be associated with further significant variation, but substantial research findings here are scarce. Generally, minority ethnic households seek positively to pursue their own individual housing strategies (just as other groups do), and vary widely in their ability to achieve their preferred outcomes in line with the specific barriers they face, and their resources and commitments. The development of a 'minority ethnic middle class' is associated with reduced social exclusion, including the choice of a degree of suburbanisation (Phillips, 1998; Harrison with Phillips, 2003). It is probable that this might be more marked for some minority ethnic, religious or age groups than for others. Nonetheless, there is likely to be a degree of socioeconomic differentiation within most communities, and perhaps the emergence or confirmation of a 'familiar social class gradient' for some housing conditions (see Ratcliffe, 1997, p 143, with regard to central heating). Each minority ethnic group has not only its own specific settlement geography but also its own potential for internal socioeconomic polarisation. The varying characteristics of households are also crucial within, as well as between, communities. There are housing implications from the higher proportions of female-headed, lone-parent families among Black people and the more extended household structures among the South Asian groups. Expected growth in numbers of elders raises significant accommodation and support issues for the future. While it has often been argued that there is a strong need for large family dwellings in particular communities, there also may well be an increasing demand for specific accommodation for elders or for smaller households in years to come. Emergent or hidden needs may exist within those communities about which, in other respects, much is already known. For example, only sparse information seems to be readily available about South Asian women who have become isolated from their communities, or for elders who can no longer call on the extended family for support.

Continuing patterns of disadvantage

Patterns of disadvantage persist across differing communities, with black and minority ethnic (BME) groups still tending to be relatively poorly housed. Housing difficulties sit alongside other difficulties. In comparison to their representation in the population, people from minority ethnic communities are more likely than others to live in deprived areas, to be poor, to suffer ill-health, and to live in overcrowded housing (Cabinet Office, 2000, p 17). Local housing needs studies have reinforced the evidence of disadvantage for specific minority communities, highlighting large proportions of people with long-term illness or impairment, or noting effects of practical problems such as inability to use central heating fully because of high costs (Ratcliffe, 1996b; Gidley et al, 1999). Particular groups in specific urban localities have extremely low incomes and limited housing choices. Platt and Noble (1999), referring to Birmingham, confirm impressions of severe poverty for Bangladeshi, African-

Caribbean/Black–Other and Pakistani groups, and include the observation that "we can calculate that 56 per cent of all Bangladeshi children under the age of 16 are living in poverty" (Platt and Noble, 1999, pp 20-3). Pakistani and Bangladeshi people seem to be in very deprived housing conditions, with both groups being affected by high levels of overcrowding, and with many in 1991 having no central heating (see Ratcliffe, 1997, pp 141-3).

Although it is desirable to bear in mind local market conditions and the choices available to particular groups of households when considering tenure patterns and preferences, low-income home ownership persists as an important feature of black and minority ethnic experience generally. Social rented housing is also very significant. Movement into the latter tends to reflect low incomes, but household characteristics should be kept in mind also, and we have already touched upon the significance of such housing for women (Peach and Byron, 1993, 1994; Phillips, 1996). As far as 'down-market' owner-occupation is concerned, this could sometimes be problematic for owners where repair and maintenance costs were high, conventional mortgages hard to obtain, neighbourhood environmental quality unsatisfactory, or property values insecure. Owner-occupier status on its own can be very unreliable when taken as a pointer to satisfactory housing experience or quality (see Harrison with Davis, 2001, p 147). Furthermore, discriminatory practices and racist harassment can have ongoing housing effects even for those who are achieving a measure of upward mobility.

One useful indicator of continuing housing disadvantage is homelessness. Reviews of local needs studies and homelessness reports and commentaries suggest that black and minority ethnic communities have disproportionately high overall rates of homelessness. However, there are differences between minority ethnic groups in the extent and nature of the experience (Chahal, 1999b; Burrows, 1997, p 57). Although London has high concentrations of homeless households, the phenomenon is not confined to the capital. Sodhi et al (2001) state that studies on homelessness show "that BME communities have disproportionately high rates of homelessness and this is clear in the case of African Caribbeans, Asians and the Irish" (2001, p 4), although for Asians we might expect homelessness to be less 'visible'.

A point sometimes highlighted is the significance of 'hidden' (or perhaps more accurately 'unrecognised') homelessness. In reviewing minority ethnic homelessness for the National Health Service Executive (London), Chahal (1999b, p 1) explains that minority ethnic homelessness "is less about street homelessness and much more about being hidden". Thus minority ethnic people "tend to use friends and relatives much more than white people" (1999b, p 1). In another study, Davies et al (1996) found some difficulty in contacting homeless young Asian people. This may have been a reflection of reluctance on the part of Asian communities to recognise that youth homelessness was a significant problem, and an insistence that whatever homelessness existed was dealt with by and within the community (Davies et al, 1996, p 6). Some minority ethnic homeless people may be reluctant to use white-run institutions, to share facilities with white clients, or to expose themselves to violence, police contact, or racist harassment through being visible 'on the street'. Services are sometimes perceived as unwelcoming, and are seen to lack black minority ethnic staff or management, or to be insensitive to cultural needs. Although homelessness manifests itself as a visible single event to which an urgent reply appears essential, it is the tip of a bigger 'iceberg' of complex housing pathway events. Thus it may point to a shortage of readily accessible social rented housing, and reflect the weak labour market positions and limited accommodation options open to specific groups (for an overview see Harrison, 1999).

Residential segregation and concentration

As Chapter Three of this volume demonstrates, there is a high degree of geographical concentration of the minorities in housing areas within parts of urban England. However, geographical concentration in itself does not necessarily indicate or cause 'social exclusion' or multiple disadvantage. Unfortunately, observers sometimes takes a simplistic view that refers to supposed 'ghettoisation', without acknowledging the positive dimensions of minority ethnic experience or the merits of living in proximity to people of similar culture and language. A ghetto should probably be understood to be something surrounded by obstacles that make it difficult to leave, or where residents find it hard to become included in wider societal networks and opportunities should they so wish. Seen in this way, a ghetto is about restrictions on people's strategies rather than implying population concentration alone. While there are some features of minority ethnic areas of residence that suggest fairly systematic exclusion from a more prosperous mainstream, this is an incomplete and very varied process. Nationally, some black and minority ethnic households (particularly Indian) are relocating in outer urban areas of better-quality housing (for analysis by Phillips of suburbanisation processes and changing ethnic geographies, see Harrison with Phillips, 2003). Thus, there has been outward movement, including some selective settlement into higher-status property outside 'deprived areas', albeit characterised by "new nodes of ethnic minority concentration" (Phillips and Karn, 1992, p 358). Furthermore, processes of what we might term local cultural, community or political inclusion within inner urban areas (often facilitated through affiliations linked to ethnicity) might be much preferred by residents to those cultural processes occurring in some outlying low-income white estates. Indeed, one hypothesis is that processes of localised 'community integration' in inner-city areas are associated with better health and well-being for minorities, and could influence a range of satisfactions and experiences, generating positive health effects among other outcomes. Certainly, it is desirable to be cautious about some recent criticism made of the separation of groups, offered on grounds that spatial separation interferes with so-called 'community cohesion'.

In any event, although many black minority ethnic people would like improved housing conditions, they frequently favour areas of existing settlement, and wish to avoid harassment and isolation that may arise in other types of locality. This is not to deny that there are many aspects of life in inner-city areas (and perhaps sometimes this includes segregated living) that are at the very least involuntary, or carry costs. A 'traditional' (and useful) way of viewing segregation and concentration in particular neighbourhoods was to think in terms of interactions between constraints and choices. On the one hand, researchers had shown how discriminatory housing provider practices in the public sector helped create or confirm segregation, while economic disadvantage and negative discrimination limited areas of successful housing search in private markets. Thus, households had faced severe constraints. On the other hand, positive reasons for clustering could include cultural, kinship and religious ties, security, or culturally relevant services and retailing.

In practical terms, households may continue to be disadvantaged by limitations of opportunities that can accompany life in inner-city areas (such as overcrowding, difficulties in obtaining insurance, reasonable housing finance or good jobs, limited access to preferred schools, or dilapidated housing). Many minority ethnic owner-occupiers are located very firmly in the lower end of the tenure in terms of property quality. The issue of ethnic penalties noted earlier can be considered in relation to inner areas. One interpretation would be that barriers to outward movement and choice of dwellings could affect even those who are prospering, via the impact of harassment and insecurity arising in some outer areas. Thus, one aspect of shared experiences across ethnic and socioeconomic categories is continuing exposure to harassment and violence. Racist incidents have both immediate and long-term effects on individuals, families and communities, and can influence people's choices of housing and localities. Meanwhile, living in poorly resourced localities and difficult environments brings financial and physical penalties alongside some potential social and safety gains.

With greater understanding of the pervasiveness of racist harassment, the negative forces restricting households' geographical housing search have become more fully acknowledged. Despite diversity, racist harassment continues to generate barriers to movement for people from many minority communities. The issue of 'no go' areas has been noted by observers, as well as the particular risks faced by black people living outside the main areas of settlement. Recently, Chahal and Julienne (1999) have summarised the extent and limitations of previous work and available data, and presented findings from their own study, which involved research in four areas across the UK. Their report examines the impact of racist victimisation on black and minority ethnic people's daily lives from their own perspectives, and touches on the strategies that families and individuals adopt to prevent or lessen racist victimisation. From the more general literature, it seems that harassment associated with residence remains widespread (albeit difficult to quantify precisely or to compare across places and studies). Chahal and Julienne summarise criticisms made in earlier studies about the inadequacy of official responses, noting the negative effects on household choice (including transfer to other, more segregated, neighbourhoods).

An additional point to stress is that spatial separation is to some degree a product of a differentiated and complex structure of preferences across groups, and is not solely (or necessarily mainly) a consequence of decisions among minority ethnic households. Many (although by no means all) white households have been more able to put their preferences into practice, moving to areas they perceive as being of better quality or higher status. A key issue for most households is likely to concern the degree of genuine and low-risk choice open to them. Policy makers need to keep this in mind, rather than leaning towards the temptations of trying to engineer social change in the expectation of being able to produce a more integrated pattern of residence.

Housing needs, disability, age and gender

There have been numerous local studies of black minority ethnic housing needs and allied topics in recent years, enriching the understanding that policy makers, researchers and local communities have of housing problems. The studies have highlighted both the diverse needs of the different communities and the commonality of housing experiences across some groups. For instance, it has been confirmed that Chinese and Asian communities appear to be experiencing changes in family structure and there may be susceptibility to "social isolation because of language difficulties", yet that all communities share the "desire to live in areas where there are other members of their community and cultural and religious facilities close by" (Sodhi et al, 2001, p 4). This becomes particularly important in later life. There are income and affordability problems affecting housing, and "access problems in terms of social housing" (Sodhi et al, 2001, pp 4-5), particularly among the Asian and Chinese. For these communities, overcrowding and housing conditions may exacerbate health problems.

Local research relating to housing conditions has frequently considered circumstances for specific groups or categories (such as elders), and calls are often made for more such work focused on particular types of households (for instance in relation to women within particular communities, or people with specific impairments). Issues of cultural needs have been identified. Some types of households certainly may have rather particular housing experiences or requirements, or may perceive the treatment that they have received as differing in unpleasant ways from that received by other people. Disability, age and gender are potentially important in these respects as far as 'race' and housing are concerned. Studies tackling minority ethnic housing needs have noted the importance of disability or chronic illness, and the question arises as to whether this has been adequately responded to by housing providers. Hard data are scarce here, although Law (1996, pp 101, 106) noted from a Leeds study that minority ethnic households remained underrepresented among those households with medical priority, and that a low percentage of minority ethnic households received disabled facilities grants. Begum (1992), in research touching on housing while covering Asian disabled people, highlights the "dual impact of race and disability", often placing people in a unique, and "particularly disadvantaged position" (1992, p 13). Zarb and Oliver (JRF, 1993b) found that older disabled people from black minority ethnic communities were more likely than their white counterparts to face problems such as extreme isolation and very low incomes, while a London report suggests considerable need for sheltered bed spaces, very sheltered units, aids, adaptations and residential care among Asian elders (Sandhu, 1998).

Stereotypes relating to 'race' or ethnicity have been important, and have meant that practitioners might overestimate the preparedness of service users' relatives and social networks to provide informal care, and "could be particularly insensitive to members of minority ethnic communities" (JRF, 1993a, p 1). Lack of explicit demand for a service may be taken wrongly to imply lack of need, ignoring the possibility that problems of information, communications or the cultural insensitivity of provision may have diminished take-up. In any event, at present there is underprovision of culturally sensitive services for some groups, and neglect of problems experienced by minority ethnic disabled people. Radia (1996) conducted a study on housing and mental healthcare needs that illustrates key problems. Radia looked at Asian people in Brent, Ealing, Harrow and Tower Hamlets. Asian mental health service users experienced problems of inappropriate housing, difficulties with neighbours, burglaries, racist attacks or harassment, and fears for their personal safety (Radia, 1996, p 1). Users did not have enough support, or the right kind of support, to be able to take charge of their own lives, and services were not culturally sensitive to their needs (and did not cater for those not fluent in spoken or written English). Interviewees did not think that there were community services that were suitable or adequate, or that catered for what they really required. Among strategies for change, Radia (1996, pp 2, 22-5) suggests offering:

- a range of quality, supported independent housing and residential care;
- · specialist housing catering for the needs of Asian people with mental healthcare problems;
- trained outreach support workers to service both residential projects and those people living more independently in the community.

A substantial number of reports have focused specifically on elders, and Chahal and Temple (2000) have recently systematically reviewed the research position here. A key conclusion of their overview report is that different minority ethnic communities have differing and changing expectations about both service provision and the changing structures of family life. Yet the whole area of aspirations and expectations of older people from minority ethnic groups is largely unexplored. Chahal and Temple add that there is no evidence of work being undertaken with younger groups about their future demands on the housing markets (2000, p 1). Perhaps this is surprising in view of the anticipated rapid increase in numbers in pensionable age groups, but researchers do sometimes include within their coverage people coming up to retirement. We would argue that thought should certainly be given to the future implications that differing tenure patterns and access to resources will have for types of demand and need in specific places, taking into account changing expectations and practices within communities. The predicted steep increase in numbers of elders within certain communities, coupled with an altered ratio of younger to older people, is likely to enlarge the demand for community services, and may diminish the potential for households to arrange informal care (for a brief commentary on relevant research, see Tomlins, 1999, pp 9-10). Factors likely to make forms of accommodation appeal to elders will include a low risk of harassment, culturally sensitive staffing, outreach or support services, respect shown for people, intelligent design that takes culture into account, proximity to family, safety from crime, and closeness to community, shops and places of worship. Chahal and Temple (2000, p 1) highlight the paucity of research on older people from minority ethnic backgrounds and mental health needs and abuse. They also indicate that minority ethnic people need to be discussed as individual groups, and in fact as individuals in their own right, with very different needs and experiences.

A good illustration of the complications surrounding provision for elders is available in work by Karn et al (1999). In Manchester, they found that the needs and preferences of elders were rather different for each ethnic group studied. For instance, the "degree of stress on independent living and on family care varied considerably", as did "views on forms of residential care" (Karn et al, 1999, p 131). The African-Caribbean informants emphasised independence, and had positive views of sheltered housing, although they found inadequate cultural sensitivity in the way specific sheltered schemes were currently run. By contrast, the South Asian group in this research "scarcely mentioned independence" (p 132), and for them it appeared that good domiciliary services and flexible forms of housing (allowing older and younger generations to live with or near each other) were likely to be most effective. Yet there was evidence that overcrowding put severe strain on arrangements for families caring for their own elders, and dissatisfaction with current arrangements "included the elders themselves" who sought greater space and privacy (Karn et al, 1999, p 132). Karn et al observe that adaptation of their own (or family's) homes is "the model most likely to meet the needs of all but the most frail or isolated" (1999, p 132). They indicate that (given a shortage of larger dwellings) acquisition and allocation of adjacent properties might be useful, perhaps with consideration given to options such as a connecting door, or simply members of an extended family living next door to each other (1999, p 134).

For women from black and minority ethnic communities, observers have often drawn attention to:

- problems of unacknowledged (or 'hidden') homelessness coupled with reliance on temporary accommodation from family or friends;

- lack of geographical choice or satisfactory provider responses in social renting;
- isolation or stigma associated with separation from families, partners or communities;
- difficulties in private markets because of low incomes;
- adverse housing outcomes linked to domestic violence or abuse. (See Gill, 2002, pp 167-71, for a summary regarding homelessness.)

Gender is significant for lifestyles and housing outcomes, and clearly intersects with other variables (age, ethnicity, and so forth) to give complex patterns. Disadvantage is experienced by female heads of household, whether single persons or heads of families. Phillips (1996) has observed that male heads of household in three broad ethnic groups (white, Indian and Black Caribbean) are significantly more likely to own property than female heads, and less likely to be represented in the local authority sector (see also Peach and Byron, 1993; Phillips, 1997, p 175). Even for South Asian groups with high ownership rates overall, the public sector "features significantly" when the household is female-headed (Ratcliffe, 1997, p 135). Interestingly, the heads of tenant households of black minority ethnic-run Registered Social Landlords (RSLs) are more likely to be women than are RSL tenants as a whole. (RSLs include most important housing associations.) More new lettings are in any case being made to women than to men across the RSL sector (Lemos and Crane, nd, pp 1, 5-6), although it is difficult to explain these findings without detailed enquiries. What is certain is that there is often relative disadvantage for women on several dimensions. For instance, Phillips (1996, p 64) found that Indian and Black Caribbean female heads of households were more likely to be living in terraced housing than were the male heads of households within their own ethnic group.

When women leave their partners, there can be severe problems. Rai and Thiara (1997, p 9) remark that black women often face "the dual problem of racism from the wider society and rejection from their own communities".

Strategies and preferences

Along with increasing recognition of diversity has come greater acknowledgement that different households or groups of households may have varying expectations, preferences and housing strategies. Information about whether past choices were constrained can be illuminating. A good example is Third et al's (1997) study of owner-occupiers in Scotland, where 25% of minority ethnic respondents said that they would have preferred an alternative tenure at the time they entered owner-occupation (1997, p vii). Such findings might appear to run somewhat against the grain of most recent information on preferences, which has tended to show the long-term wish for owner-occupancy, and has sometimes coupled it with the concept of social rented housing having in effect a 'negative utility' for particular groups. The answer is that caution is required on expressed tenure preferences, which may be amended or revised in the light of specific circumstances, and could change over time. Without some indications about pathways and resources, statements are difficult to interpret. For instance, it has sometimes been thought that African-Caribbean households might not attach stigma to council housing in the way that is often felt to occur for Asian households, and that social rented housing is perceived as a valuable and necessary service. Yet, for some African-Caribbean households, entry to this housing might form part of a longer-term strategy aimed at purchasing a house at a feasible cost (although differentiating effects of family/ household structures on tenure opportunities within this minority ethnic group should not be overlooked)[1].

Housing experiences, achievements and strategies may vary not only over lifetimes, but also between cohorts of migrants or generations of settled groups. It is possible that 'ethnic penalties' and market conditions shift, and that upward mobility or assimilation have significant effects for some groups more than others. There may be generational as well as ethnic group differences in propensity to migrate out of established areas of settlement. On the one hand, younger households might be less determined in their preference for a 'traditional' locale, while on the other hand, youth unemployment might constrain or slow spatial dispersal in some places. At the same time, the boundaries between groups may become blurred through the increased numbers of households with mixed ethnic origins. When looking at household needs and trajectories, it is important not only to include new or less visible groups, but also to be aware of distinctions between cohorts.

Policy issues and ways forward

This chapter concludes with a brief comment on the performance of social rented housing, and on what is known in relation to one specific governmental policy preoccupation in particular: the functions of such housing in relation to the outward movement of minority ethnic households.

Many of the 'classic' housing and 'race' studies of the past dealt directly with the performance of housing organisations in terms of 'racial' equality. In particular, several widely known reports clearly demonstrated negative discriminatory practices in council housing allocation processes (Simpson, 1981; CRE, 1984, 1988; Phillips, 1986; Henderson and Karn, 1987; Sarre et al, 1989). In recent years, the emphases of research have altered, as housing associations and The Housing Corporation have taken centre stage, and as the cultural sensitivity of services has moved up the agenda, as well as because equal opportunities expectations have become more widely established (with consequent efforts to improve practice). Nonetheless, although overt racisms are less evident in social rented housing work today, research continues to cast doubt on the effectiveness of RSLs on several fronts[2]. The proportion of RSLs' lettings to black minority ethnic households actually fell through the 1990s, from 14.4% in 1990-91 to 12.7% in 1998-99. The percentage of lettings to Irish and South Asian households did not even match their representation in the population, despite a general acknowledgement that minority communities are frequently experiencing severe housing problems. More of RSLs' total lettings activity had been occurring in local authorities with a below-average black and minority ethnic population in 1998-99 than in 1990-91 (Tomlins et al, 2001, pp 14-15, 27).

It is hard to tell how far particular categories of tenants or potential tenants still face limitations on housing choice, because of discriminatory attitudes, crude stereotypes, investment priorities, or assumptions by managers about where minority ethnic tenants will feel safe or comfortable. There may be minority ethnic groups established in social renting who face difficulties in moving to better-quality estates, but there is little information about recent trends affecting the locational options of specific groups (such as homeless people, female-headed households or small, newer minorities). Furthermore, the picture in areas of strong demand (where tenancy turnover may be low) needs researching. Little is known about the quality of service provided to specific kinds of households by social rented housing landlords.

One important debate about practical policy options focuses on the issue of movement into more peripheral areas, and on possibilities for overcoming barriers to entry to social rented housing estates outside existing areas of minority settlement. Social rented housing may be increasingly available in some localities where demand has been falling, while minority ethnic households (particularly from some Asian communities) are living not far away in low-quality, older private sector dwellings with severe problems of poverty and overcrowding. Yet take-up of new council tenancies among some minority groups is slow. While at least some minority ethnic households have a strong desire to move out of inner-city areas, barriers may be perceived in terms of the absence of other minority ethnic households and associated facilities and shops, as well as in the form of potential harassment (see Birmingham City Council, 1998, p i). Along with responding to direct experiences of harassment, black minority ethnic households may wish to distance themselves from what they perceive as a crime-prone, less respectable and 'rough' (generally white) estate culture, just as many white people would wish to do. Bowes et al (1998) capture the tone of thinking well in the title of their report: *Too white, too rough, and too many problems*. More attractive white estates that might suit some minority households may well be located further from core areas of settlement, and present problems because of having few existing black tenants. Housing association accommodation may have a better image than some council housing (especially when managed by black and minority ethnic housing associations), but there may be few substantial appropriate geographical 'outliers' or nodes of development away from established settlement. Black and minority ethnic-run housing associations attract minority ethnic tenants, but have limited stocks of dwellings, and may possess few outlying estates. Furthermore, relatively high rents and perceived limitations on the long-term availability of the right to buy may deter potential tenants from approaching housing associations in general. Some RSLs may be reluctant to develop new schemes (with minority ethnic tenants in mind) away from 'traditional' areas of settlement. There are concerns about anticipated problems of racist abuse, harassment and violence from the local white population, which could undermine the commitment of minority ethnic tenants and create management problems (Robinson, 2002, p 101).

A good overview of key issues is provided by Phillips and Unsworth (2002), who note an ambivalence about clustering in the traditional areas of minority settlement that may affect younger people in particular. Their study involved a national survey of local authority housing departments and housing associations operating in 14 urban localities, and looked at the priority given to widening ethnic choice, the strategies developed, implementation and success. As they put it, there is a need for sensitive and well-tuned policies to support minority ethnic households now wishing to move to non-traditional areas within the social rented sector. They reveal that some housing providers have begun implementing strategies of creating "settlement nodes" or clusters in more outlying areas, perhaps underpinned by inter-agency initiatives and tenant support (Phillips and Unsworth, 2002, p 85). We might argue that elements tailored to community needs and preferences could include conversions to create larger dwellings (or reconversions of subdivided properties), and opportunities for low-cost home ownership. For social renting, there might be potential in some towns for black minority ethnic block housing allocations or large targeted shares of tenancies, linked with management and ownership structures facilitating involvement of black-run collective or representative housing organisations (whether within independent or federal organisational structures). Who controls property assets and management on estates is potentially a significant matter for households and communities. Ways of overcoming barriers suggested in Birmingham have included improving housing-related services, supporting provision of cultural and religious amenities, providing 'race' awareness training for outer-area residents, and providing better public transport links to inner-city locations (Birmingham City Council, 1998, pp i-ii; compare Karn et al, 1999, p 8). The Bradford report, *Breaking down the barriers* (Ratcliffe et al, 2001, p 32), lists various actions which in the longer term might help to increase access to the outer estates. These include:

- improving the standard and cultural sensitivity of service delivery;
- more joined-up policy making between organisations;
- developing appropriate property types/sizes, including houses for shared ownership and outright sale;
- information provision;
- developing community support networks;
- aiming for linked lettings where families are rehoused together to improve security;
- exploring the "potential role of BME housing associations".

One feasible strategy in the short term is seen as possibly increasing access to housing locations between the more congested urban areas of central Bradford and the outer estates.

Programmes encouraging minority ethnic households into areas of existing white settlement are unlikely to be straightforward, even with supportive community development strategies. There is wide variation in the available information about preferences, and there are locally differing implications from ongoing events such as stock transfers, development of common housing registers, recent innovations in approaches to choice and allocations, and organisational change. Nonetheless, as the Bradford study confirms, although owner-occupation is the dominant aspiration of many groups, this should not mean overlooking the significant potential roles of social renting in a period when new households face financial constraints and difficulties in obtaining adequate dwellings in 'traditional' areas of settlement (see Ratcliffe et al, 2001, p 8). Whether as a transitional option or a longer-term tenure destination, social rented housing may be becoming more significant. We do not have a good up-to-date picture of the extent and character of demand from within specific minority ethnic communities for social rented tenancies. In some places, expressed demand might already be high relative to the capacity of housing providers to meet it by offering tenancies in preferred or acceptable areas. The conclusion that social rented housing is important, however, does not mean forgetting the roles played by private housing markets (and the significance of governmental policies related to these), or the potential for collective forms of ownership such as co-ops and self-builds. At present, policy levers remain rather limited as far as 'down-market' owner-occupation and its sustainability are concerned, while the collective ownership dimension remains underdeveloped.

Notes

[1] For relevant comments, see Karn et al (1999, p 58); Law et al (1996, pp 39-40); also Peach and Byron (1993).

[2] See especially Somerville et al (2000); Tomlins et al (2001); Robinson et al (2002).

EIGHT

'All the women are white, all the blacks are men – but some of us are brave': mapping the consequences of invisibility for black and minority ethnic women in Britain[1]

Heidi Safia Mirza

Slipping through the 'racial equality' cracks

The uncompromising recommendations of the Stephen Lawrence Inquiry[2] with regard to institutional racism generated widespread political and public response and commitment to racial equality. However, in their efforts to avoid being labelled as institutionally racist, few organisations reflected on the gendered nature of their racial equality policies and practices. Few have stopped to consider that the Lawrence Inquiry was an all-male committee and may therefore have had a male-centred view of racism. In terms of racial equality, it is still a man's world. Thirty years on, the African-American women's saying of the 1970s – "all the women are white and all the blacks are men, but some of us are brave" – still holds true (Hull et al, 1982). Gender is still seen as a white woman's issue, while it is taken for granted that 'race' is a black male issue. Black and minority ethnic women appear to fall into the cracks between the two. They are often invisible, occupying a 'blind spot' in mainstream policy and research studies that talk about women on the one hand or ethnic minorities on the other.

Black and minority ethnic women still do not seem to be part of the race equality picture of the new millennium. The 'new language' of racial equality and inclusion, in the context of the liberal democratic discourse on equality and anti-discrimination, has been constructed around the dominant masculine agenda of objectives and targets, enforcement and evaluation, recruitment and audit (CRE, 2001). The pervasive discourse on social inclusion through 'respecting diversity and achieving equality' has at its core the concept of the 'recognition of difference'. However, the social construction of 'difference' does not include the invisible or messy contradictions black women pose by their presence. Diversity is now about good public relations and inclusivity as good business sense (Fredman, 2002): it is more about 'getting the right people for the job on merit' and the 'business benefits of a more diverse workforce' (Cabinet Office, 2001). It is not, then, about removing exclusionary barriers to participation and equal access. However, when we read of the commitment of public sector organisations to 'meeting needs', 'facilitating access', 'flexibility', 'embracing difference', and 'working in partnership' with black and minority ethnic people (Cabinet Office 2002), it is assumed that racial equality and social exclusion are gender-neutral experiences.

It could be argued that persistent inequalities and patterns of social exclusion among black and minority ethnic communities are being addressed universally through new and far-reaching anti-discrimination and equalities legislation. Recently the 2000 Race Relations (Amendment) Act, the 1998 Human Rights Act and the 2000 EU Employment and Race Directives have widened anti-discrimination, equal treatment and positive provision (Hepple et al, 2000; Fredman, 2002, DTI, 2002b). Protection now can cover direct and indirect discrimination based on sex, race, colour, language, religion, political or other opinion, national or social origin, association with a national minority, property, birth, racial or ethnic origin, religion or belief, disability, age and sexual orientation. Such extensive protection needs to be accessible to the most marginal and excluded people in order to be credible. However, the covert nature of the process of exclusion experienced by black and minority ethnic women challenges the context of these legal and institutional mechanisms for redressing inequalities.

In spite of progressive equality legislation and the move toward a single equality commission, it has been demonstrated that black and minority ethnic women are still categorised in unmeaningful ways in the application of the legislation. These women are often simplistically 'objectified' in terms of preconceived political and social categories that often underpin social policy and equalities thinking. Women's life experiences of poverty, neglect, marginalisation and discrimination are disaggregated in official documentation and statistics in terms of being either women (and hence 'gendered') or ethnic minorities (and hence 'raced'). Such 'intersectionality' (Crenshaw, 1993; UN, 2000), which characterises the equality discourse, artificially dichtomises racial, gendered and other identities when, in effect, each one is experienced through the other (Brah, 1996)[3].

> [R]acism and sexism are interlocking systems of domination that uphold
> each other. It does not make sense to analyse 'race' and gender as if they
> constitute discrete systems of power. (Maynard, 1994, p 21)

As a consequence of 'intersectionality', black and minority ethnic women fall between the scope of the separate legislative provision for race, sex and disability discrimination. Black and minority ethnic women who experience complex interacting levels of discrimination have been found to suffer 'double' or even 'triple jeopardy' (Bradley, 2001). They are very rarely able to make multiple discrimination claims based on the holistic nature of their racialised/sexualised being and experience (Gregory, 2002). In effect, a gap remains between policy and legislation on one hand, and experience and practice on the other. At the heart of this gap is the lived reality of black and minority ethnic women.

Scoping the issues: multiple identities and lived realities

Before we can explore gender inequalities and differences in any meaningful way, it is important to establish that black and minority ethnic women are *holistic individuals*. Like everyone else they have complex multiple identities. When we consider their daily lived realities, they express their subjective identity in the collective gendered terms of familial roles and responsibilities as mothers, workers and wives (Mohanty, 1997). They talk about duty to the family, protecting their children, surviving poor conditions, caring for others and organising for change. They express themselves as active agents – as 'feminised beings'.

The distinctive demographic characteristics of black and minority ethnic women are often hidden within the broad brush of census classifications, which masks the diverse economic, social, cultural and religious differences between and among the 2.3 million black and minority ethnic women living in the UK (WEU, 2002a). The generalised census categories tell us that, in Britain, South Asian women make up the largest group within the category 'black and minority ethnic women', with 22% of Indian descent, 15% of Pakistani and 6% of Bangladeshi origin. Black–Caribbean women make up 13% and Black–African 12%. In addition, 12% of black and minority ethnic women are classified as Mixed, 6% as Other–Asian, Chinese women make up 4%, Black–Other 2%, and Other 8%[4].

Few research and statistical studies have explored the social and cultural positioning of black and minority ethnic women (Mirza and Rollock, 2001). Important differences are overlooked when women are subsumed under the homogenous term 'black and minority ethnic women'. This overarching collective term can incorporate a range of identities, from recent refugees fleeing war and famine, to third-generation African-Caribbean settled migrants, who have established work and cultural patterns in the UK. The issues become even more complex when we look further within, to reveal the multiple identities of the various black and minority ethnic women. The women have multiple experiences in terms of age, sexuality, disability, religious and cultural differences. For example, an older Asian woman who has worked in the family business and is widowed will have a very different identity, and face different equality issues to a young Somali mother who is a doctor yet as a refugee is unable to secure employment. Each woman therefore has a different 'story' to tell. Just as their experiences are different, so, too, have multiple definitions of themselves evolved in terms of their everyday lived experience of gendered and racialised social relations (Brah, 1996; Mirza, 1997a).

Universalistic generalisations concerning the majority (white) female population do not hold true for different black and minority ethnic women. For example, all minority ethnic groups contain more children and fewer elderly people than the white population. Thus, while child dependency ratios for Bangladeshi women are more than double that of the white population, elderly dependency ratios are three times lower for black groups than for white (CRE, 2002a; WEU, 2002b). Similarly, Pakistani and Bangladeshi women are more likely than white women to have children in their early 20s, be married and not working (Bhavnani, 1994; Bhopal, 1998; Dale, et al, 2002). In contrast, African-Caribbean women are more likely to be employed in skilled manual work and are three times more likely to be lone parents than any other group (Owen, 1994; Berthoud, 2001). Thus, the issues faced by different groups of women in terms of caring, working, health and service needs are substantively different, and therefore have implications for equality of access.

Mapping the 'race/gender gap'

As an exercise, mapping gaps in 'race' and gender research can be very revealing. It shows patterns of visibility and invisibility that can be described in terms of the 'normative absence/pathological presence' couplet that characterises much of the research in this area (Phoenix, 2001). In studies based on such diverse fields as family, work, education, health, community participation, law, rights and representation, black and minority ethnic women are either excluded from mainstream 'normative' (white) analysis, or included as negative 'pathological' problematic (black) subjects.

Families of (wo)man? Black and minority ethnic women as mothers, wives and carers

Much of the research on black and minority ethnic families is still characterised by a normative absence/pathological presence approach. Black and minority ethnic families are often omitted when normalised, unproblematic issues are being studied, such the government's 'work–life balance' campaign, but included and focussed on when issues are constructed as problematic, such as teenage pregnancy (Phoenix, 1996; Berthoud, 2001). Few studies of black and minority ethnic British families have moved beyond attempts to explain how and why they differ from white ethnic groups in terms of structure and values.

Attempts to provide understandings of black and minority ethnic women's own discourses of familial care mirrors mainstream feminist preoccupations with the 'hidden private domestic sphere'. The focus of such research includes:

- cultural and religious practices;
- intergenerational kinship structures;
- childcare and other ways of mothering;
- marriage and (lone) parenthood[5].

While it is important to explore familial patterns and reveal the domestic context of oppressive cultural and religious practices within the 'private sphere of the home', the implications of 'lifting the veil' to open up and examine the inner dynamics of familial life among 'other' cultural groups needs to be clearly thought through (*The Guardian*, 2001b).

In the absence of a balanced research agenda that centres upon women's own voices, such an emphasis on 'cultural difference' within familial structures can reinforce stereotypical cultural perceptions of certain groups through a process of 'objectification of the other' (Simmonds, 1997). Revealing the consequences of patriarchal familial structures that oppress and silence women can also lead to problematic images of black and minority ethnic women as either disempowered victims or overempowered matriarchs. Stereotypes of 'docile Muslim daughters forced into arranged marriages' (Brah, 1996) or 'overbearing black African-Caribbean "superwomen" who marginalise their men' (Reynolds, 1997) prevail in our everyday culturally racialised and deeply sexualised perceptions. Issues of power and agency in women's lives are rarely considered.

Families, then, are far more complex that is assumed in much public discourse. While there are clearly different types of familial structures among cultural groups, this is often mediated by individual situations and specific social and geographical locations. Nevertheless, limited or rigid inter-ethnic knowledge about black and minority ethnic families and parenting has often lead to racialised constructions with policy – and hence personal – consequences for black and minority ethnic women. While African-Caribbean mothers have often been seen as inadequate (Reynolds, 1997; Lewis, 2000), Asian mothers are often seen as too controlling (Parmar, 1982; CCCS, 1982). However, surprising differences between different ethnic groups in terms of forms of household organisation subvert gender expectations and stereotypes. For example, many Muslims and Sikhs favour the paid employment of married women outside the home (Bhachu, 1991; Brah, 1996).

Research shows that minority ethnic families – like all types of families – are not static: rather, they change over time (Modood et al, 1997). In response to living in Britain, women negotiate cultural practices that have previously been taken for granted. Thus, an understanding of the diversity of family forms within black and minority ethnic families can illuminate the ways in which society is changing. For example, one of the most significant changes shaping the 'new' multicultural landscape of Britain is the rapid increase in 'mixed race' marriages and children of mixed heritage (Phoenix and Owen, 1996; Ifekwunigwe, 1999).

Other familial patterns, such as the high rates of lone motherhood among African-Caribbean women, are now being mirrored in the white community, where there are sharply rising trends (Berthoud, 2000b). Although matriarchal familial arrangements such as single mothers have been deemed a negative social construction in mainstream familial (patriarchal) discourse, they have social and cultural relevance and meaning in different historical and economic times (Mirza, 1992). As Reynolds (1997) argues, lone motherhood in black families does not mean pathological disadvantage. Lone mothering encompasses a range of ways in which absent fathers contributed to their children's lives. Just as lone mothering (a positive cultural choice) reflects economic change, so too does the impact of globalisation and movement of peoples affect familial relationships for minority ethnic women in Britain. Chamberlain (1999) argues that lateral relationships of siblings, uncles and aunts are of more importance culturally and economically than conjugal relationships for Caribbean transnational families.

Relatively little is known about black and minority ethnic familial patterns and change. However, even less is known about 'taboo' subjects in difficult-to-access, research-sensitive areas – familial rape and abuse, domestic violence, suicide, drugs and alcohol – although community projects and refuges exist to support women in need[6]. In the Home Office, there is little sympathy for black and Asian women as victims of domestic violence. Southall Black Sisters has campaigned long and hard to show how women are either deported when their marriages break down or imprisoned with unbelievably harsh sentences when they go against the grain and try to fight back in self-defence (Patel, 1997). However, in many cases, black and Asian women are caught in the conflict of not telling the authorities about their ordeals for fear of racist reprisals such as deportation or the loss of their children.

Working against the odds: black and minority ethnic women and labour market participation

Many generalised 'normative' assumptions are made when we talk about 'women's employment in Britain'. Under this blanket term, black and minority ethnic women's specific circumstances remain hidden. However, it is well established that Black African and Caribbean women are more likely to be in full-time work, and work longer hours, than white women are. Economic activity also varies greatly between minority ethnic groups. While seven out of 10 Black–Caribbean and white women are active in the labour market, this is true of only two out of 10 Pakistani and Bangladeshi women. The social class structure of black and minority ethnic women is much more concentrated in the intermediate and skilled non-manual groups, except for South Asian women, who are most likely to be in the partly skilled class (Bhavnani, 1994; WEU, 2002b).

On the surface, it is easy to claim that "given the very low rates of Bangladeshi women in the workforce, it is not meaningful to analyse their socio-economic position in any depth" (Eade et al,1996, p 156). This belies the hidden fact that Pakistani and Bangladeshi women, and refugee women, are often undocumented workers in unregulated areas of the informal economy such as homeworking, and can face disproportionate discrimination from employers (Dale et al, 2001, 2002).

In a similar gendered oversight, little emphasis has been placed on the specific circumstances of young black and minority ethnic women in programmes such as New Deal for Work (BLMN, 1998). Rates of unemployment among black and Asian young women aged 16-24 are much higher than young white women and as high as those among young black and Asian men (Modood et al, 1997; CRE, 2002a). Such a gap in equality is considered a crucial future flashpoint in terms of 'social cohesion' for young black and Asian men (Cantle, 2001; Ousley, 2001). Yet, few consider in any depth the social and economic consequences of this growing gendered/racial divide for second-generation black and minority ethnic young women. Studies of black and minority ethnic young women show their active participation in the redefinition of their feminised identity through music, dance and acts of transgression (Weekes, 1997;Walter, 1999). Clearly, they have an important role to play in 'multicultural' social change (*The Guardian*, 2001a).

Release from family commitments is a real issue for all minority ethnic women who want to work. As a consequence of the government's modernising agenda, there is a commitment to double the numbers of black and ethnic minorities in the public sector by 2005 (Cabinet Office, 2002). However, to achieve these ambitious recruitment targets, it is important to recognise that racial equality is a deeply gendered issue. In order for black and Asian women to get into senior levels in the public sector, their particular childcare needs must be recognised (Cabinet Office, 2003). However, it is difficult to obtain statistics on the numbers of black and Asian women, as figures are compiled by *either* ethnicity *or* gender (see Cabinet Office, 2002). There are figures on ethnicity and on women – but not both at the same time. In the few cases where employers cross-reference race by gender, the picture is bleak. In a post-Stephen Lawrence Inquiry recruitment drive, London's Metropolitan Police estimated that there were just 900 black police officers. Fifteen per cent of those are minority ethnic women; none in the senior levels. Numbering just 135 in total, women are rare. A great deal more is expected of them as young recruits in a city where the minority ethnic population is one and half million[7].

Similarly, the army's antiracist strategy appears to exclude a positive vision for a black female role at a leadership level. In a statement on the army's drive toward racial equality, General Sir Charles Guthrie celebrated black figures such as Colin Powell, then chairman of the US Joint Chiefs of Staff, and the one unnamed black British male military leader in Kosovo. However, he overlooked the hidden armies of black women that cook, clean and service them[8]. Zero tolerance of humiliating racist male initiation rites in macho work environments such as the police and the army is vital, but it should not overshadow the very real problem of black female harassment in the workplace. A recent survey revealed that, in our 'respectable and genteel' university system, minority women are twice as likely to experience racial harassment as minority men (Carter et al, 1999).

Role models and mentoring schemes to 'raise up and let in' the marginal and excluded appears to be the dominant British strategy for achieving racial equality in the workplace. They aim to build confidence, develop self-esteem and establish facilitating networks (Appiah, 2001). Such schemes realistically recognise the need for 'bridging social capital'; that is, 'informal' social networks that link black and minority ethnic people to white employers (Heath and Yu, 2001). However, mentoring programmes such as the CRE's 'Visible Women' campaign have limited effect in the context of structural workplace issues such as discrimination, unequal pay and workplace harassment, which disproportionately affect black and minority ethnic women at all levels, including the visible professions (Bhavnani and Coyle, 2000). No amount of inspirational role models or strategic mentoring schemes will change ingrained patterns of structural inequality and hidden privilege (CRE, 1996).

In the face of postmodern global change, the British Civil Service (which has traditionally recruited disproportionately from Oxbridge, notably to higher status positions and to some departments), is still engulfed in the meritocratic moral debate for and against anti-discrimination and positive action for black and minority ethnic people (Puwar, 2001). In the context of ambitious and unrealistic recruitment targets, ethnic minorities are warned 'they will only get there on merit' and 'not to raise their expectations too high' (Mirza, 1999a). Yet, despite merit, motivation, and self-confidence, demonstrated by their commitment to work and education, black and Asian women are the least represented of any group in senior posts. Overall, in universities, government, schools and hospitals, black and minority ethnic men are more likely to be in professional and managerial positions (Modood et al, 1997; Cabinet Office, 2002b).

Explaining educational inequality: success and failure for black and minority ethnic women

Research shows that black and minority ethnic young women experience underachievement and suffer disproportionate levels of exclusion in relation to the white school population (Gillborn and Mirza, 2000; Osler et al, 2002). However, as the girls' overall performance is better than the boys, they are often overlooked when the effects of institutional educational inequality are tracked. Girls attain rather higher grades than their male peers, but the gender gap within their groups is insufficient to close the pronounced inequality of attainment suffered by their ethnic group as a whole. For example Bangladeshi, Pakistani and African-Caribbean girls not only experience inequalities of attainment by comparison with white and Indian girls, they are also less likely to attain five higher-grade GCSEs than white and Indian boys. Thus, not only are there ethnic inequalities between groups of pupils of the same sex but also some consistent and significant inequalities of attainment *between* ethnic groups regardless of pupils' gender.

However, comparisons of different ethnic groups and genders in terms of educational outcomes must be treated with caution. In our desire to celebrate multiple identities and diversity, a postmodern construction of difference has emerged that has the potential to embed creeping forms of benign racialisation.

A 'new racism' is evolving where groups defined in terms of their race and sex are hierarchically compared and contrasted with each other on the basis of their inherent cultural capacities, 'natural' talent, genetic ability and IQ (Mirza, 1998; Gillborn and Youdell, 2000). Such racialised constructions of comparative difference among different ethnic and cultural groups dominate common-sense political thinking.

Qualitative research shows how accounts of educational success and failure become 'racialised' through culturalist explanations. African-Caribbean girls doing relatively well in comparison with their white male and female peers within the locality of their schools has been much cited as evidence of gendered strategies to resist oppression and overcome racism. These strategies are located simplistically in fixed essentialist constructions of 'strong black female role models'. Unlike males, it is believed that black females can overcome disadvantage by drawing on their 'matriarchal roots'. This culturalist explanation of black female success ignores the wider structural context of gendered and racialised patterns of migration, labour market opportunities, and patterns of sexualised racism in the educational system (Mirza, 1992, 1997b). Given these explanations, the relative success of black girls has generally been misinterpreted to mean that only black boys and not girls face inequality (Mirza, 1999b). Hence the key issue in the Department for Education and Skills (DfES) is the 'inclusion' of black boys against a background of their educational underachievement, high rates of truancy and disproportionate levels of exclusion.

Just as black African-Caribbean girls' educational success is culturally constructed, so too are Indian girls' achievements. Whereas for black girls explanations are framed in terms of their 'maternal role models', for Indian girls it is their parents' 'positive orientation to educational values' that are valorised. Cultural orientation is expressed as a 'racial' fact. Educational success is constructed as inherent to that gendered/racialised group. Little account is given of the relatively privileged social class background of the majority of this migrant group. Little is said about the geographical areas where pockets of working-class Indian pupils do the least well in terms of not achieving five or more higher-grade GCSEs (Gillborn and Gipps, 1996; Gillborn and Mirza, 2000). In contrast to other minorities who 'fail', Indians are deemed a 'model minority', held up as an example to us all of the power of personal and cultural transcendence and the impossibility of there being any institutional racism.

Institutional racism can manifest itself in many forms. Despite the government's funding of faith schools, our knowledge of the experience of Muslim girls is limited (Brah and Minhas, 1985; Basit, 1997; Haw, 1998; *The Guardian*, 2001a). Though teachers give anecdotal evidence, there appears to be an official 'conspiracy of silence' around the 'disappearance' of significant numbers of young Asian women from school when they reach puberty. Such issues rock the multicultural boat, which fails to champion the human rights of young Asian women in the face of patriarchal community leaders with fundamentalist mantras around religious rights (Patel, 1997). Such stories do not seem to capture the public imagination like the black and Asian male story of criminalisation that preoccupies the media daily. Women only appear as voiceless victims in faraway lands (as in the case of Cherie Blair's championing of Afghani women in the face of the Taliban).

Levels of participation in further and higher education are as high among black and Indian women as among white women (both 23%). However, only 7% of Pakistani and Bangladeshi women have further and higher qualifications (Dale et al, 2001, 2002; WEU, 2002b). Research shows that, regardless of qualifications, ethnic minorities pay 'ethnic penalties' in the job market (see Chapters Two and Five of this volume; Berthoud, 2000a; Heath and Yu, 2001; Cabinet Office, 2003). Despite qualifications, only a few minority ethnic women attain the status of managers or professionals. Only 4% of African-Caribbean women, 3% of Indian and 7% of Pakistani women are in the professional and managerial class, compared with 21% white women. In a wasted pool of human resources, it appears that black and minority ethnic women are still locked into low-status women's work, reach the glass ceiling for promotion, and experience twice as high levels of graduate unemployment (Carter et al, 1999).

However, black and minority ethnic women's commitment to education remains unshaken. They invest not only in their education but also in the education of their children. African-Caribbean women are involved in setting up Saturday schools, community schools run by and for the black community (Reay and Mirza, 1997). Minority ethnic women teach in African, Muslim and Turkish schools at weekends and through the holidays, even at the cost of their own health and well-being, to ensure that their children – who are being failed by mainstream schools – do well. It has been argued that such evidence of educational urgency and collective action among black African-Caribbean women deserves recognition as a 'new social movement' (Mirza and Reay, 2000a). In contrast to masculinised accounts of social change that valorise riots and visible clashes on the streets, the invisible, quiet, conformist but collective acts of mothers as educators can be seen as acts of resistance given the context of racism and discrimination. In creating 'black' alternative worlds, with different meanings and shared 'ways of knowing', the women's active agency is ultimately far more subversive and transformative than that expressed through male clamour.

'Other ways of knowing': black and minority women, community participation and activism

Black and minority women are either absent or marginal in key reports on urban regeneration and partnership strategies. Yet, as research has shown, black and minority ethnic women are involved in capacity building at the grassroots level. Black and minority ethnic women, including Muslim women, have been active in campaigning for equality at the local level (Sahgal and Yuval-Davis, 1992; Patel, 1997). Although black and minority ethnic women are diverse in terms of culture, religion, age, length of residence and type of entry to the UK, they nevertheless share a similar social positioning – that is, "marginalised from the loci of power" (Thorogood, 1989, p 331). Although hidden from view, black and minority ethnic women do organise collectively and effectively. As Sudbury (1998), Davis and Cooke (2002) and Mirza and Reay (2000b) demonstrate, black and minority ethnic women's organisations are grassroots, organic and built on women's ability to develop affective relationships with each other, with friends and with neighbours. Such emotional and social capital demonstrates women's collective agency through invisible and undervalued acts of caring, 'giving back' and personal accountability.

Research documenting black and minority ethnic women's narratives when confronting the education and health services tells about being strong, brave, clever and dignified in the face of others' perceptions of them as strange, stupid, manipulative or voiceless victims (Mirza and Reay, 2000b; Mirza and Sheridan, 2003). The strategies that black and minority ethnic women employ to change their localities, neighbourhoods and schools, are not simply 'coping strategies', but are grounded in self-actualisation and 'real knowledge', derived from their lived realities of racial and gender exclusion (Mirza and Reay, 2000b). Such real knowledge, or 'other ways of knowing', are based in ideologies of resistance in which the women evolve identities of refusal. They do not accept the dominant discourse but redefine their world with their own codes, values and understandings (Mirza, 1997b). In opposition to popular constructions of them as feckless, disengaged and alienated, many women tell stories of the creative and inventive strategies they use to preserve cultural dignity. In the context of limited access to rights, many women talk of cultural strategies they have evolved to 'fight for their rights'. They construct proud and brave identities as 'natural survivors' and ' challengers of injustice'. Ultimately, they know this means they are seen as problematic in the 'system'. As Phoenix (2001) points out, by living in a racist society, women develop practices that allow them to co-exist with different world views, while keeping their alternative identity and spirituality intact.

Despite women forming the 'backbone' of their communities (*The Guardian*, 2001a), gender is not part of the racial equality agenda. Social exclusion strategies, urban renewal and community regeneration are seen as gender blind (SEU, 1998). But how can we rebuild our neglected inner cities without black and Asian women's participation? After all, they are the 'heart of the community' and that should make them the starting point (Bryan et al, 1985). Black women know what it takes to be effective and inclusive. They are the embodiment of the 'third way'. They have been engaged in strategic joined-up thinking to combat racism in their lives long before the government adopted it. Making black and minority ethnic women a key constituent of local community action and leadership is essential to changing race relations (Brownill and Drake, 1998). However, issues around isolation, community safety and racial victimisation are emphasised by black and minority ethnic women as essential to their participation and inclusion (Chahal and Julienne, 1999).

Getting in and getting heard: access to health and well-being for black and minority ethnic women

Strategies to achieve equality and access to health services for women form the subject of many reports (Nazroo, 1997; Acheson, 1998; King's Fund, 2001). However, there is a need for closer links with black and minority service users and more sophisticated analysis of the different health needs of women without pathologising communities. One example is the overriding association of African women with HIV and Aids (Hammonds, 1997), or Asian women with self-harm and suicide (Nazroo, 2002).

A recent study of black and minority ethnic women's health issues showed their conditions were seen as a consequence of either cultural practices or ethnic 'predispositions' to certain illnesses or conditions (Mirza and Sheridan, 2003). In the study, the women were universally seen as 'a problem'. There was a crude cultural reductionism that underpinned this way of thinking. It was the women's 'difference', in terms of language, diet and ways of childcare, that framed how they were perceived in the healthcare system. Many Asian and refugee women were pathologised as 'complainers' and dismissed (often with a 'pill') as a nuisance by doctors. However, it was the women's gendered and racialised social positioning that made them vulnerable or feel unwell, often sending them into spirals of depression. Ironically, in the discourse on 'respecting diversity' in the health service, the women's 'cultural problems' were also seen as the solution. Access to language and changing the women's diets were the main focus of 'good practice' rather than organisational change or institutional reflexivity.

Similarly, the black African-Caribbean women, who were positioned differently from the Asian and refugee women as workers in the health service, experienced a comparable underlying process of racism and construction of their difference. At work, the processes of institutional racism within the organisations positioned them as unambitious, difficult, or just invisible because of their identities as survivors or maternal duties as breadwinners. As a consequence, they were often not promoted or were excluded.

Positive change in the women's lives was articulated through their own narratives of agency, self-determination and ways of working around the systems of exclusion. Their strategies included their own folk knowledge, self-help and community solutions. Their strategies served to mirror that which was lacking in the health services. Their cultural ways were not problems but strengths. However, such creativity and self-help was neither valued nor developed in the health service, which operated a top-down approach to equalities. The official language of inclusion, with its discourse on difference, flexibility and community partnership, was juxtaposed with a contradictory practice of targets, audits and enforcement.

From incarceration to asylum: rights, representation and the law

While anti-discrimination legislation is now well established, our equalities agencies – such as trade unions, the Equal Opportunities Commission (EOC), and Commission for Racial Equality – need to acknowledge issues around differential access to those rights for black and minority ethnic women. Despite the public preoccupation with the 'black male mugger and drug dealer', it is black and Asian women who are the most overrepresented group (in relation to their population size) in the prison system. In a country where minorities make up just 7.5% of the total population, 24% of female prisoners are minority ethnic women, and 17% minority ethnic men (CRE, 2002b).

Black and minority ethnic women are also serving disproportionately long sentences. Little is known about the effects of incarceration on familial relations and mental well-being among black and minority ethnic women. White male judges mete out disproportionately harsh custodial sentences to black and Asian women, who are seen as not behaving as they should (Kennedy, 1993). In our criminal justice system, black and Asian male violence against women is often deemed culturally acceptable and sanctioned. Zoora Shah, who has been imprisoned for 20 years for killing her abuser, had her case for appeal dismissed as the court decreed her story of self-defence was "not capable of belief" (Southall Black Sisters, 1998). Despite claims of being a 'mature multicultural society', there is still a liberal reluctance to get involved in other people's cultural matters for fear of being called a racist. Such latent collective social inaction means pandering to outdated cultural practices of 'colourful and ethnic' patriarchal religious communities, which undermine women's individual human rights.

In a knee-jerk reaction to the death of Stephen Lawrence, the Metropolitan Police are working with an idea of 'race hate' crime as something mainly experienced by young male youths on the street. For them, race hate is not about the complex, hidden ways that black women are sexualised, harassed or raped by men of other cultures. In a recent case, a group of white male youths were sexually and racially abusing Asian young women on a bus. When the Asian conductor intervened, the boys assaulted him. The subsequent court case dealt with the racist male assault. The sexual racialised violence suffered by the young women went unremarked: they just dropped out of the picture (Mirza, 1999a).

Gender-related aspects of asylum claims and, in particular, an understanding of gender-related persecution need to be integrated into the Home Office determination process (Crawley, 2001). Although women and their dependants flee persecution, immigration and asylum policy assumes that the model refugee is male, articulate, and a member of a political group. However, women are often engaged in dangerous unofficial political activity, providing shelter and food for dissidents. The male bias inherent in the rules of the asylum and immigration system means they often cannot qualify on their own terms – only their husband's. Sometimes women seek sanctuary as they are sexually violated or forced to marry. But the burden of proof is so onerous or humiliating that women will face death or incarceration rather than be publicly shamed (FCO, 2000).

Since September 11, there has been a significant growth of interest of Muslim women in the press[9]. As Spivak (1988, p 297) says, it is the work of the postcolonial feminist to ask the simple question "what does this mean? – and begin to plot a history". When we do so, what is revealed is a pattern of eurocentric universalism and cultural relativism (Mohanty, 2000). This pattern goes back 30 years to the debates of the 1970s on Third World women and sexual reproduction (Carby, 1982); the 1980s debates on female genital mutilation (El Saadawi, 1980); and 1990s debates on black female sexual harassment (Morrision, 1993).

When Muslim and black women appear and (disappear) in the media, it is as others wish them to – white feminists champion them as the docile wife, or the exploited worker. A complex life becomes a blank slate waiting to be inscribed with meaning by those who wish to gaze upon the Muslim female and 'name' her. In a reappropriation of the Muslim female's agency, she is the object (not the subject) of her story. In a postmodern reworking of the racialised 'colonial gaze' where, in the past, "white men save brown women from brown men" (Spivak, 1988, p 297), we now have white women (and men) saving Muslim women from Muslim men. While patriarchal atrocities and acts of violence are to be challenged in no uncertain terms, black and Third World feminists have taken issue with the cultural superiority and simplistic, sensationalised cultural constructions that negate black female identity and agency, and depolitise their (embodied) struggles for self-determination.

Carving out a 'third space': mapping black and minority ethnic women's struggle for recognition

The invisibility of black women speaks of the separate narrative constructions of race, gender and class: in a racial discourse, where the subject is male; in a gendered discourse, where the subject is white; and a class discourse, where race has no place (Mirza, 1997a, p 4).

It is almost a cliché to say black and minority ethnic women have been 'left out', 'could not be found', or 'could not be incorporated' in research studies. Minority ethnic women appear to occupy a 'blind spot' where they are often overlooked in 'normative' mainstream analysis.

Black and minority ethnic women are absent from many key reports and studies on ethnic minorities[10]. As ' bearers of the races' and 'guardians of culture' (Yuval-Davis, 1993; Brah, 1996; Alexander and Mohanty, 1997), women are deemed central to the ideological construction and reproduction of national identity and hence the (multicultural) state. However, in the Commission on the Future of Multi-Ethnic Britain (Runnymede Trust, 2000), black and minority ethnic women only get a three-page mention in the 314-page report. The new multicultural vision of 'Britishness' is made up of gender-neutral ethnic 'communities'. The inclusive 'national story' they propose 'writes out' the complexities of a gendered/racialised struggle for a women's place in the postcolonial national picture.

Similarly, minority ethnic women are not given inclusive consideration in key policy research on women. The stated policy of the EOC is that "ethnicity is not usually included, only when feasible to do so"[11]. And again, the Cabinet Office Women's National Commission report, *Future female – A 21st century gender perspective* (WNC, 2000), outlines 'working with diversity' as an aim, but proceeds to discuss women's issues in education and the labour market with the implicit assumption that they are white and homogenous. In an otherwise upbeat document, Asian women are reflected in a small downbeat section on double disadvantage of sexism and racism. Black–African and African-Caribbean women are absent from the ethnic analysis. The same standards that apply to gender mainstreaming in research policy and political practice should also apply to ethnicity and social exclusion. With regard to the invisibility and marginalisation of black and minority ethnic women in research and official documentation, we are starting from a low baseline of practice. There is a need to move toward establishing an ethical and ideological position to include sensitivity toward gendered racialisation. A checklist for gender/ethnic mainstreaming[12] and gender/ethnic proofing and awareness[13] would enable us to see new dimensions in social issues.

When included in studies, black women and minority ethnic women are so often inappropriately positioned as members of the passively constructed 'socially excluded'. However, in opposition to this, new forms of engagement have emerged as black and minority ethnic women, who are defined and excluded through their gendered racialisation, adjust their strategies to accommodate a changing variety of racially contested public and private spaces (Hill Collins, 1998). These 'acts of citizenship', which require 'other ways of knowing', are rarely given legitimacy in the classical political and social discourse on citizenship and belonging that underpin the current debates on social exclusion. As mothers, wives and workers, their agency and activism sheds new light on traditional conceptualisations of citizenship. In their gendered/racialised version of citizenship, the women combine their social capital and emotional capital skills of resourcefulness and networking, enabling them to become collective transformative agents. Their activism and radical forms of 'giving back' open up a third space of strategic engagement (Mirza and Reay, 2000b). This third space has hitherto remained invisible as the traditional gaze on the public (male) and private (female) dichotomy in current citizenship theory has obscured 'other ways of knowing' and thus 'other ways of being' a citizen.

Partnership, capacity building and development work with key community and women's organisations would help develop a grounded, positive approach to social exclusion and racial equality. As 'invisible' transformative agents, black and minority ethnic women deserve to be recognised as the 'new' citizens in theory, policy and practice. From the evidence of this chapter, it seems that recognition of their intrinsic value may be some time away. In the meantime, we hold on to hope, and adopt the chant of our transatlantic sisters:

All the women are white, all the blacks are men – but some of us are brave!

Notes

[1] For this chapter, I have used the popular and 'official' terms 'black' and minority ethnic women. This is not a term women tend to use themselves, and there is much controversy about what it really signifies and to whom (Modood et al, 2002). It has evolved due to the complex and political nature of racial definitions. In the social construction of identity it is argued that there is no scientific or biological foundation for racial difference. Thus 'black' is not a 'race'/racial category, but a politically contested homogenous term that has come to mean those who are visibly and politically racialised as 'other'. It has been appropriated positively by some groups, such as 'black' African-Caribbean women and politicised British non-white women, to enable them to identify themselves (Brah, 1996; Mirza, 1997a). Ethnicity, on the other hand, includes self-defining religious and cultural groups, who can be similarly racialised as culturally defined groups. However, because of differential power among and between ethnic groups, inherent differences in worth may not necessarily apply in the same way as with 'black' groups (Cornell and Hartmann, 1998; Runnymede Trust, 2000). However, while those defined as 'ethnic' make up majority populations globally, they find themselves defined as small 'minority' migrant communities in the UK – hence the term 'ethnic minority'. In response to this, many now prefer the term 'minority ethnic'.

[2] In 1993, Stephen Lawrence, a 17-year-old young man of African Caribbean heritage, was stabbed and killed in a racial attack while waiting for a bus in South London. The white youths who killed him were never brought to trial. The report into the police handling of the crime (Macpherson, 1999) had 70 recommendations in areas as diverse as education and employment, recruitment and family liaison.

[3] Gayatri Spivak calls the erasure of women from official discourse a form of 'epistemic violence' (Spivak, 1988). In her study of Sati, the self-immolation (suicide by burning) of widows in colonial India, Spivak argues for a 'dubious' understanding of the women's individual agency and expression of free will at the moment of immolation. In the context of the laws of Hindu patriarchy and colonial rule, the Indian woman "disappears in subject constitution (law) and object formation (repression) ... not into pristine nothingness ... but into a violent shuttling which the displaced figuration of the 'third world woman' is caught between tradition and modernisation ... to mark her (the sexed female subject) disappearance with something other than silence and non-existence, a violent aporia between subject and object status" (Spivak, 1988, p 306). It could be argued, in a similar deconstruction, that the 'black' woman in 21st-century Britain, framed between the two patriarchal and postcolonial discourses of racial equality and gender equality, exists in a vacuum of erasure and contradiction (Mirza, 1997a).

[4] However, the statistical categories do not necessarily give us a clear picture of women in multi-ethnic Britain. White ethnic groups, such as Irish, Southern and Eastern Europeans, are often subsumed under White. Turkish and Middle Eastern communities are classified as Asian–Other, while significant new migrant and refugee communities,

such as Somali are categorised as Black–Other. Similarly, new and growing identities that reflect social change and complex multiplicity among minorities in the UK are defined as Mixed Race in relation to the white majority in the 2001 Census. This analysis is from the Labour Force Survey (Spring 2002), Office for National Statistics, as 2001 Census data disaggregated by sex and ethnicity were not available at the time of writing (March 2003).

[5] For examples of qualitative research on cultural and religious practices, see Westwood and Bhachu (1988); Afshar (1994); Brah (1996). For intergenerational kinship structures, see Berrington et al (1994); Chamberlain et al (1999). For childcare and other ways of mothering, see Chamba et al (1999); Reynolds (1999); CAVA (2000). For marriage and (lone) parenthood, see Edwards (1994); Woollett et al (1993). Quantitative analysis of minority ethnic families reveals a diversity of familial patterns and structure (Berthoud and Beishon, 1997; Berthoud, 2000b).

[6] See, for example, groups such as Southall Black Sisters, Newham Asian Women's Project, Manningham Housing Association, the Black Women's Support Project, Birmingham Mosque (*The Guardian*, 2001b). However, these exist on very limited funding and struggle to obtain legitimacy from mainstream charitable funders (Davis and Cooke, 2002).

[7] Reported at the national 'Into Leadership: Diversity in Britain in the 21st century' Conference, London (23 June 1999). See Mirza (1999a) for an analysis.

[8] Also reported at the national 'Into Leadership: Diversity in Britain in the 21st century' Conference, London (23 June 1999). See Mirza (1999a) for an analysis..

[9] 'Behind the Burka' (Polly Toynbee, in *The Guardian*, 28 September 2001); 'Barefaced resistance: women of Afghanistan (Natasha Walter, in *The Guardian*, 20 July 2002); 'The other side of the veil: what women say about Islam' (*The Guardian*, 8 December 2001).

[10] For example, recent research on 'ethnic minorities and pension decisions' concludes that the inclusion of women would make an "unduly complex piece of research" (Nesbitt and Neary, 2001, p 94).

[11] This statement was made by the EOC in response to a telephone enquiry for the Joseph Rowntree Foundation "Researching black and ethnic minority women" (Mirza and Rollock, 2001). Similarly, the Office for National Statistics was unable to supply detailed specific breakdowns by gender and ethnicity, saying this is not "normally required". This upset the black female researcher – she experienced this as personal negation and erasure from the public discourse.

[12] Mainstreaming equality through meeting statutory requirements and enforcing the law is but one half of the equation. While auditing and monitoring, action plans and performance targets are all tools of achieving this, truly embedding equality is about promoting equality through changing cultural practice by "building issues of equality

into policies and practices across a broad front, taking account of all the equality strands" (DTI, 2002a, p 10). Mainstreaming in this sense means engendering reflexive organisational change through the "process of assessing the implications for different individuals of any planned action including legislation, policies and programmes, in all areas and at all levels" (Runnymede Trust, 2000, p 286).

[13] See *A checklist for gender proofing research* (www.eoc.org.uk).

NINE

Police lore and community disorder: diversity in the criminal justice system[1]

Virinder S. Kalra

Introduction

This volume has so far traced patterns of ethnic disadvantage as they are experienced in a number of aspects of life in modern Britain. A number of key themes are evident. First, it is possible to identify both continuities and significant changes in patterns of advantage and disadvantage, within and between groups. Second, the key role of socioeconomic status, or class, has been revealed on a number of occasions. Third, despite the evidence of upward social mobility for members of at least some minority ethnic groups, persistent evidence remains of an 'ethnic penalty' mediated by discrimination and racism.

In this chapter, the focus changes somewhat to an aspect of the lives of Britain's minority ethnic population that relates not simply to material well-being in its various guises but to what is in some ways a more intangible question: the experience of a sense of full, substantive citizenship. Nowhere is such a sense more palpable than in relations with key state institutions, and few such institutions can be said to have had such a consistently significant impact than the criminal justice system as a whole, and the police in particular. This is not to say that socioeconomic status is irrelevant to experience of the criminal justice system. There is a long history of research demonstrating the significance of class for the patterning of recorded crime and for the organisation of policing. What will be argued in this chapter, however, is that ethnicity mediates experiences of the criminal justice system in specific ways, and that the police play a key role in shaping that mediation. A key mechanism, this chapter argues, is the process by which differential ethnic marking of groups takes place in and through the process of policing. It will also be argued that there are both continuities and changes in the way this process has developed over recent years. In particular, we shall see that the fact that the criminal justice system operates differentially on different racialised groups with different effects is not a new feature of the way that law and order is implemented in Britain.

Indeed, the civic disturbances that marked a number of England's northern towns in mid-2001 were evidence of a continuing differential marking of populations. However, a novel feature of that marking process concerns the shift of target from African-Caribbean to Asian Muslim males. Anecdotally, the situation prior to the 1990s could be described in terms of African-Caribbean men being marked out for the over-zealous application of the law and police activity, as demonstrated by statistics on 'Stop and Search', arrests and prison population. By contrast, Asians were marked by an under-zealous application of the law, marked by low levels of arrest for racial intimidation and attack perpetrated against them. This crude set of distinctions serves to illustrate that diverse outcomes have long been a reality for different racialised groups in Britain when engaging with the criminal justice system.

Were it accepted that discrimination operates differentially, then, rather than talk about racism in the singular, we need to think about racisms. This is the logical extension of thinking about groups in terms of diversity. When different groups have different experiences of interacting with the criminal justice system, then different processes of racialisation must be at play to result in positive or negative outcomes. This means that the same institution can treat different groups in different ways and that particular policies have a role in the creation and maintenance of ethnically marked difference and therefore ethnically marked advantage and disadvantage. We shall see in due course how a process of this kind resulted in the effective creation of distinct ethnicities through the specificities of local policing. This represents a particular manifestation of the process of ethnic boundary creation and maintenance discussed in Chapter Two of this volume. For the moment we need to set the stage by considering the evidence of differential outcomes in the criminal justice system, particularly in relation to sentencing and the prison population.

Diversity in the operation of the criminal justice system

The mass of quantitative evidence showing discrimination in the workings of the criminal justice system has been growing since the 1970s. There is a considerable body of academic and policy literature that points to many discrepancies at all stages of the workings of the various aspects of the law[2]. An analysis of the workings of the police, judiciary and prison service shows a consistent pattern of differential treatment. Following the 1991 Criminal Justice Act, the Home Office has been obliged to collect information that can help to tackle discrimination in the performance of the criminal justice system. Perhaps the most comprehensive collation of statistics in this regard has been published in *Statistics on race and the criminal justice system 2000* (Home Office, 2000). A summary of some of the main findings of this document illustrates the extent to which the criminal justice system works differentially in terms of both ethnicity and gender. We begin by looking at the prison population.

Table 9.1 shows that African and African-Caribbean males and females are highly overrepresented in the prison population when compared to the general

Table 9.1: Prison population by ethnicity, nationality and gender (1999)

Ethnic group	All nationalities, males	British nationality, males	All nationalities, females	British nationality, females
White	81.5	85.7	75.3	84.8
Black	12	10.2	19	11.9
African	2	1.1	2.7	0.8
Caribbean	7.1	6.3	9.9	5.7
Other	2.8	2.8	6.4	5.4
Asian	3.1	2.3	1.1	0.7
Bangladeshi	0.3	0.1	0.1	0.1
Indian	1.1	0.8	0.4	0.3
Pakistani	1.7	1.3	0.5	0.3
Other	3.4	1.8	4.5	2.4
Chinese	0.1	0	0.2	0
Other–Asian	1.4	1	0.5	0.4
Other	1.9	0.8	3.8	2
Not known	0	0	0.1	0.1

Source: Home Office (2000)

population of England and Wales (British nationals aged 15-64). Thus, while 95% of this population are white, 1% black, 3% South Asian, and 1% other ethnic groups, black males constituted 12% of the prison population and black females a shocking 19%. Even when measured against 1991 Census data, which included those who were not British nationals, the overrepresentation of black groups is stark. The data are complicated by the fact that the Home Office distinguishes between foreign nationals and British minority ethnic groups. Since a large proportion of those categorised as 'ethnic' are foreign nationals – 4,490 (30%) males and 680 (5%) females at the end of January 2002 – this tends to inflate the proportion of prisoners from minority ethnic groups as compared with the general population. However, we should also note in the context of the distinction between British and foreign 'ethnics' that a considerable number of settlers of South Asian origin (that is, those with rights to stay in Britain) have not taken up nationality.

The prison population has remained quite stable over the period 1994-99 in terms of ethnic composition despite an increase in the overall population of prisoners. The only notable increase has been from Asian groups, and this has mainly come from an increase in Pakistani males (Home Office, 2000).

Perhaps following the diversity agenda ahead of many other government departments, the Home Office also considers religious difference in its monitoring of prison populations. In 2000, Christian denominations made up the majority of the prison population (57%), with 7% of the population from the Islamic faith. Statistics provided in the report *The prison population in*

2000 (Elkins and Olagundoye, 2001) give a detailed breakdown of the prison population by ethnic group and religion, covering a large range of faiths, from Buddhist through to those with no religion. The results of the 2001 Census on religious populations indicate that the number of Muslims in prison far outweighs their presence in the general population (3.1-4%). This is in contrast to the Sikh population, whose prison representation is in proportion to its population (0.7%), and the Hindu population, which is underrepresented. It should also be remembered that these religious populations do not map directly on to ethnic group, especially in the case of Muslims, where the majority is from a black ethnic group (Elkins and Olagundoye, 2001).

Even when foreign nationals are excluded, the patterns of overrepresentation characteristic of the prison population have given rise to a long-running debate about the impact of ethnicity on criminal offences. In particular, a recurrent theme is the question of whether rates of criminality among Black Caribbean and African populations are greater than among the majority population. The key debate is between those who argue that the criminal justice system treats minority ethnic groups differentially and those who maintain that certain minority ethnic groups are more likely to offend. Statistics are often used to show that criminality is greater among the black population and low among the Asian population. However, statistics also show that crime rates are highest among urban populations and among the young, both factors that apply to black and minority ethnic (BME) populations. Perhaps of more concern is the fact that, even before statistics were collected, the association of young Black Caribbean people with crime was used a political tool to mobilise against immigration (Hall et al, 1978; Solomos, 1989). In the most recent analysis of the statistics, Bowling and Phillips (2002, p 106) conclude, using self-reporting studies by offenders, that the volume of offending echoes "the official view of 30 years ago that the African/Caribbean crime rate is much the same as that of the 'white' population and that the rate for Asians is much lower". More critically, the whole question of conceiving of the object of 'black crime' as an area of empirical research is problematic given the political reality of the way in which it has been constructed as a tool for talking about race relations in Britain (Keith, 1993). Indeed, it may only be by the reconfiguration of the notion of criminality that any accurate relationship between ethnicity and offending may emerge.

The perpetuation of the official view on African-Caribbean offending is one example of institutional racism in the workings of the criminal justice system. The prison population also highlights the fact that this works differentially to produce a situation in which certain ethnic groups are more heavily represented in that population. However, there are other issues of concern when looking at the relationship between minority groups and the criminal justice system. Perhaps of most significance when considering reasons for mistrust of the police are the incidents of 'Stop and Search' as well as the comparisons of arrests and cautions that arise from such activities.

Perhaps more than any other form of police activity, 'Stop and Search' (or SUS as it was then known) was cited as one of the key factors behind the alienation of black youth in the build-up to the 1981 and subsequent civil disturbances (Keith, 1993). More recently, under the 1984 Police and Criminal Evidence Act, police officers have the power to stop and search any person suspected of having carried out a crime or acting in a suspicious manner. This factor obviously allows for the subjective experience of officers to play a significant role in determining those whom they consider suspicious. When the perception of officers is that black people are more likely to commit crime, it also creates the conditions for a cycle of harassment (Bowling and Phillips, 2002).

The general figures on 'Stop and Search' from Home Office research once again illustrate a pattern of differential treatment. Of all stops carried out in 1999-2000, 8% were of black suspects, 4% of Asian suspects and 1% of other non-white suspects. More stark are figures for searches and arrest rates. Black people are five times more likely to be searched than white people, while the figures for Asians vary widely according to police force. The general reason for deploying 'Stop and Search' related to stolen property, though for Asian and black people 'drugs' was the most cited reason. Notably, however, the proportions of those arrested from 'Stop and Search' were 13% for white people, 17% for black people, 14% for Asians, and a further 17% for other ethnic groups also facing arrest.

In the 1981 and 1985 disturbances, the role of 'Stop and Search' activities, police perceptions of African-Caribbean criminality, and community perceptions of the police were deemed to play a key role in the events leading to civil disorder. Therefore, it is useful to compare a range of statistics from those police areas where the 2001 disturbances occurred with other areas where there are large BME populations but where no comparable events occurred. Table 9.2 gives figures on 'Stop and Search' in five police force areas, three where disturbances occurred (Greater Manchester, Lancashire and West Yorkshire) and two with high BME populations but no major disturbances.

These figures highlight, as we might expect, a higher percentage of 'Stop and Search' of the black population (relative to their presence in the general population) and about the same proportion for Asians. Indeed, it is in the non-disturbance areas of Kent and the West Midlands where the percentage of Asians stopped is higher than their proportion in the population as a whole.

Table 9.2: Percentage of 'Stop and Search' of persons (1999-2000)

Police force area	White	Black	Asian
Greater Manchester	88.8	5.5	3.3
Lancashire	93.8	1.1	3.8
West Yorkshire	87.7	4.0	9.7
West Midlands	63.0	15.4	20.2
Kent	92.0	1.2	3.0

Source: Home Office (2000)

Table 9.3: 'Stop and Search' per 1,000 population aged 10+

Police force area	White	Black	Asian	Total
Greater Manchester	22	98	19	23
Lancashire	22	67	24	22
West Yorkshire	16	49	23	16
West Midlands	8	44	21	9
Kent	27	67	75	29

Source: Home Office (2000)

Perhaps a more useful measure, given the propensity of young males to be involved in civil disorder, is the 'Stop and Search' rate per 1,000 population aged 10+.

Table 9.3 shows that there is great variation in the use of 'Stop and Search', by both areas and ethnicity, and that there is no necessary mapping of these rates onto the areas where the disturbances occurred. Although the figures for West Yorkshire do indicate markedly differential treatment of Asians and Blacks compared with the white population, this is nowhere near as significant as the figures for Kent.

As far as arrest rates are concerned, Greater Manchester and Lancashire have marginally higher rates of arrest of Asians than the whole population, whereas for West Yorkshire there is a considerable difference. Twelve per cent of white people are arrested after 'Stop and Search', whereas the rate is 16% for Asians. More useful figures would include an age profile of those arrested as this might also produce a more marked effect on Asians than on other groups, given both the demographic profile and the profile of those involved in the disturbances.

Statistics relating to age of all those arrested by ethnic group are also available. These allow us to consider whether young people (here defined as aged 10-21) are more likely to be involved in crime as a percentage of the total arrested population. As Table 9.4 shows there are no great differences in terms of Asian young people and the general population (with the exception of Lancashire). Even though in each of the areas affected by riots Asian young people are more likely than the total population to be arrested, this may be due to the younger

Table 9.4: Percentage of those arrested aged under 21 in total population and Asian population

Police force area	Asian	Total
Greater Manchester	44	43
Lancashire	45	39
West Yorkshire	40	43
West Midlands	41	45

Source: Home Office (2000)

Table 9.5: Policing in the areas of disturbance

	Bradford, Easter	Bradford, July	Burnley	Oldham
Numbers involved	100	400-500	400	500
Injuries: Police	None	326	83	2
General public	20	14	28	3
Cost of damage	£117,000	£7.5-10 million	£0.5 million	£1.4 million

Source: Denham (2001)

age profile of the population rather than a trend towards greater criminalisation. In addition, the statistics available only cover those aged under 21, whereas young people are more conventionally defined up to the age of 24 or 25. As a result of the limitations of the data, it is therefore difficult to draw reliable conclusions.

When we turn our attention from general policing patterns to consider the impact of the disorders themselves, in terms of those arrested and police injured (Table 9.5), it is clear that the main conflict, especially in Bradford, was between the police and Asian young people.

Overall, 395 people were arrested during the riots, the majority of whom were Asian young men. Sentences for those convicted have varied from three to five years for serious offences, though concerns have been expressed about the length of sentences for first-time offenders[3]. Those arrested were predominantly aged 17-26, predominantly local, and mainly of Pakistani and Bangladeshi heritage. The areas where the riots took place were also on the margins of, or otherwise near, areas occupied by Asian Muslims. Indeed, even though the causes of the riots are multiple, and the incursion of Far Right groups has been cited in all of the subsequent policy reports, ultimately the conflict in all three areas was played out between predominantly Asian Muslim young men and the local police. Clearly, the relationship between the police and sections of the young male Asian Muslim population is something that needs to be explored further. It would be expected, therefore, that the inquiries into the disturbances would shed some light on this matter. One of the key concerns of the Scarman Report (1981), following the large-scale unrest of 1981, was the relationship between the black (here African-Caribbean) community and the police, and the tense relationship between young black people and the police in particular. The differential treatment of this group by the police and the criminal justice system was identified as one of the key frustrations that led to the riots in Brixton. In contrast, the role of the police has been relatively less focused upon when considering the responses to the 2001 disturbances.

The Denham, Cantle, Oldham and Burnley inquiries

Four reports were released after the disturbances of 2001. Two were locally based and two were national in scope. The Burnley Task Force was set up after the June disturbances and was chaired by Lord Tony Clarke. It consisted of a wide range of representatives, primarily local, from the voluntary as well as the statutory sector. The report is wide-ranging, the largest of all the documents produced, and in many ways provides the most information, although with little analysis and comment. However, discussion of the role of the police in the disturbances is largely confined to complaints about their handling of drug dealers and the fact that they were unable to deal with other common social problems. Differential treatment by the police is invoked only in terms of claims that they *favour* the Asian population. For instance:

> There is a perception in the town that the police and the council fall over themselves to protect them [the Asians]. (Burnley Task Force, 2001, p 63)

This quotation appears alongside another, which argues that all people should be treated the same regardless of race. No mention is made in any of the submissions of the possible criminalisation of certain sections of the Asian population[4].

A similar story can be found in the Oldham Independent Review led by David Ritchie, a career bureaucrat. The members of this review were drawn from the national stage – local representation was non-existent on the panel. The commissioning bodies for the research were the local authority and the police authority. Neither had a member on the panel, although a former police superintendent was a member. Policing took up one chapter of the final report, but the central philosophy underpinning the approach is highlighted in the opening paragraph of that chapter:

> The Police do not create the environment in which they work, but need to influence it, reflect it and respond to its problems. (Oldham Independent Review Panel, 2001, p 41)

This approach places the police outside the society in which they are required to maintain law and order. This populist view of the police is that of an agent above society and not susceptible to its norms is generally contradicted by many of the policies on policing that have emerged from the Home Office in recent times (Bowling and Phillips, 2002). It is also difficult to sustain, as another section of the Oldham Independent Review shows. When discussing the events surrounding the release of racial incident statistics in January 2001, which indicated that white people were numerically greater victims of racial attack than Asians, the report defends the position of the then chief superintendent in releasing the figure without any context. However, it goes on to point out that, given the heightened tension in the town, the matter could have been better handled. This is a mild criticism, but at least acknowledges that the police had some role in the tension that led up to the riots. Furthermore, the recommendation that more black and Asian police officers need to be recruited by the police again indicates an acknowledgement that the police are actually much more likely to reflect the prejudices of the society in which they live, rather than be above or somehow beyond them.

Of most significance, perhaps, is the fact that the report does not mention alienation of Asian young people from the police force. This is despite the fact that in appendix 7 of the report, where the views of the people of Oldham are summarised, the attitude towards the police among the Asian community – old and young – were negative. While the report attempts to tackle the source of this distrust, it is within an overall thesis that highlights segregation as the main cause of social unrest. The role of the local authority in providing housing and education is identified as contributing to segregation, whereas the role of the police in creating and maintaining segregation is dismissed. Indeed, the whole conceptualisation of the problem in terms of segregation allows for certain institutions to sideline their responsibilities.

The two national reports following the disturbances also focus on the question of segregation through the notion of 'cohesion'. The more substantive report is *Community cohesion* (Cantle, 2001), but the more useful is *Building cohesive communities* (Denham, 2001). *Community cohesion* was chaired by Ted Cantle and the report represents an inquiry into Bradford, Burley and Oldham together with other towns with substantial minority ethnic populations that did not suffer from any disturbances. Unlike the local reports, the police are placed in the role of a key agency that can influence and generate community cohesion. Their role in the disturbances is commended, although lack of policing, toleration of drugs and allowing areas to become off limits – which in essence all relate to the criminalisation of BME young people – were identified as areas in which improvements needed to take place. A bizarre link is therefore established (one of the many that has emerged from these events) between tensions with communities and criminality. The following sentence introduces a recommendation:

> Local authorities and police authorities should establish a protocol of support and ensure that there are clear agreements in place to enable serious problems of both criminality and tensions between communities to be tackled with the strong backing of both sides. (Cantle, 2001, p 41)

Indeed, the process of criminalising BME young people who riot is a strategy that is well worn – and has been used since the 1981 disturbances as it ties in well with the other statistics discussed earlier. This strategy is both well illustrated and clearly explained in the seminal volume *Policing the crisis* (Hall et al, 1978).

Of all of the reports, the least substantial in terms of pages but perhaps the most coherent in terms of understanding was the Denham Report (Denham, 2001), which is a ministerial document outlining future strategy. This is the only report to clearly highlight failure on the part of the police when dealing with communities in these areas. One of the key issues for concern is highlighted as "weaknesses and disparity in the police response to community issues" (Denham, 2001, p 11). Indeed, the lack of confidence in the police is also further cited as a cause for concern. However, it is not surprising that the police come under most criticism in this report as the document is aimed at influencing national policy, and in many ways it defers to the local reports to tackle specific issues. However, the way in which disorder was created in these towns is precisely due to the interplay of local and national conditions. Indeed, the importance the Macpherson Inquiry and its recommendations, and the general relationship between the police and community in the context of race relations, does not feature at all in the Denham Report and is only briefly mentioned in two of the other reports. Yet it is precisely this context that provides one of the routes into understanding the disturbances. Indeed, without this background it is difficult to appreciate the role of the police, let alone attempt to embark on policy change. This is best exemplified by considering the role of the police in the lead up to the disturbances in Oldham.

Police lore and community disorder

The weight of statistical evidence illustrates the fraught nature of the relationship between young people from racialised groups and the police. In simple terms, young black people are seen as pathologically criminal, while Asian Muslims are overly involved in fraud and drugs. Statistical sophistication in the application of diversity therefore allows for the development of nuanced stereotypes. But the central conundrum remains: if heavy handed policing was partly to blame for the 1981 riots, what role did it have to play in the 2001 disturbances, when the evidence given above still shows much lower rates of criminalisation for Asian Muslims than black groups?

While the statistical data only weakly indicate an emerging pattern of criminalisation of Asian Muslim youth, recent ethnographic work (Alexander, 2000), and the few voices that are heard in the local reports into the disturbances, paint a different picture. Here, Asian Muslim young people are alienated from both the police and from 'community leadership'. Racism in education and housing, rather than segregation and poor employment opportunities, have led to a resentment that has found no other avenue (Kundnani, 2001a). So, even though the criminalisation suffered by black youth still far outweighs that of Asians, the social conditions that create resentment are largely similar to the early 1980s. It is perhaps for this reason that the police and the criminal justice system as a whole do not get criticised in the policy response following the disturbances. This is in contrast to the Scarman Report (1981) which was a response to the 1981 civil unrest. In that case, a clear correlation was drawn between the impact of policing and civil disorder. For Scarman, the riots were "essentially an outburst of anger and resentment by young black people against the police" (Scarman, 1981, p 15). No such clear connection has been made in any of the many reports following the disturbances in 2001.

Instead, the focus has been on deprived social conditions and a view of the police as outside agents acting as referees imposing regulation on communities of which they were not themselves a part. What is missing from the equation – and this is why the local reports have been disappointing – is a clearer picture of the role of the police in creating and managing the conditions for civil unrest. This presents the police as active agents in the creation of the conditions that led to the rioting, rather than as the passive recipients and controllers of social disorder created by deprivation and social poverty. A detailed consideration of the role of the police in one of the riot areas (Oldham) illustrates this point.

The relationship between the police and Asian Muslim and white ('no culture') young males is often assumed to be structurally similar. Both groups of young men maintain that the police discriminate against them. It is then possible to argue that the police are caught between these two groups, rather than having a particular institutional position in relation to the Asian Muslim youth. This places the riots firmly into the context of debates about maintaining social order. A number of commentators have also made great play of how both sets of youth had more in common with one another and that the central problem was one of thuggery (see Kundnani, 2001b, for a critique of this). Naturally, the response to this should be greater emphasis on extending police powers to tackle issues of youth criminality.

Yet it is difficult to maintain this neutral stance when examining the nature of racial incidents in Oldham. Since 1998, racial incident statistics in the Oldham area have consistently shown that, in crude terms, violence and abuse towards whites is greater than that towards minority ethnic people. Ray et al (1999), who have been researching racist violence in the Greater Manchester area, highlight the consistency of the attacks by Asians on whites, but more importantly focus our attention on the police response. The chief superintendent of Oldham, Eric Hewitt, released a press statement maintaining that "gangs of Asian young people were causing resentment in the town". This was backed by the local newspaper, which ran an article following the release of the statistics in 2001 emphasising an alleged epidemic of racist violence in Oldham. Drugs and violence were said to be at the forefront of an Oldham Asian crime crisis. There are similarities here with the 'Asian gang' crises so well documented by Alexander in her book of the same name (Alexander, 2000). Alexander's book relates to London and the East End, where, incidentally, Tower Hamlets returns similar figures on racial harassment to those in Oldham.

For the record, these crude figures say nothing about rates of violence – you are still seven times more likely to be attacked in Oldham if you are Asian – and nothing still about historic and contemporary underreporting of racial incidents, nor indeed the fact that racial incidents cover a wide range of activities from violence to person and property to name calling. When one looks at the detailed breakdown of the incidents, we find that, for the period March 2000 to March 2001 (that is, before the riots), the number of violent incidents against minority ethnic groups was almost double that against white by the minority ethnic groups.

It can be argued that the seeds of the riots were fertilised and watered by the release of raw racial harassment statistics in January 2001 that contained no mention of rates or analyses of different types of incident. Their release and the subsequent press coverage enabled the creation of a white victimology that was exploited by Far Right parties. But there is something perhaps a little deeper going on here. The application of the Macpherson definition of racist incident essentially allows the police to record any incident that involves a majority and minority ethnic person as racist. This is an accurate application of Macpherson but, as Chahal (1999a) argues, the practice goes against the spirit of the inquiry that was set up to investigate the murder of the black teenager Stephen Lawrence, and the subsequent report, which spends most of its time exposing the poor treatment of minority ethnic groups by the majority. This interpretation is not new. Indeed, it is an abbreviation of the current definition used by the Association of Chief Police Officers. However, in a letter to the *Oldham Evening Chronicle* (11 October 2001), Hewitt himself recognised that the definition is subjective in nature, and as such does not necessarily meet the test of the law in terms of racially aggravated offences. This probably helps to account for the very low conviction rate for offences of this kind (currently under 1%). However, it does create a situation in which any crime by an Asian on a white is open to interpretation as racially motivated by any of the parties concerned, including the investigating police officer.

Understanding diversity in this context requires an understanding of the processes that lead to the mobilisation and formation of collectivities that can be called 'ethnic'. It demands that we cease equating ethnicity with minority and recognise that all people have some ethnic affiliations (see Chapter Two of this volume). In the Oldham context, two ethnic groups were created in the process leading up to the riots. On the one hand, a pathological Asian Muslim male criminal, usually in a gang and, on the other, a victimised white disenfranchised, cultureless group, now publically represented by the British National Party (BNP). These two 'ethnic' groups are not those for which we have statistical information; they are not particularly owned or targeted by policy and, perhaps more importantly, not owned by the 'ethnic' groups we think we are familiar with. After the events in the north of England, respectable members the Pakistani/Kashmiri and Bangladeshi communities, elected councillors, and chairmen of mosques almost unanimously condemned the events. Few were willing to engage with the role of the police, even when condemning the role of the BNP. At the same time, the fact that a white ethnicity was successfully mobilised, not for extremist activities, but at the ballot box by the BNP, also indicates that the mainstream political parties have ignored and not been able to represent a section of the white population. In both cases, to tackle these issues there is a need to understand the local processes and mechanisms by which ethnic groups are mobilised.

In the Oldham context, it was the most mundane of matters that caused resentment, but one that illustrates an important point about cultural diversity. The Owl is the centrepiece of Oldham Borough's charter mark. It sits in the centre of the town's emblem. It was also engraved into a number of bollards in the town centre, which were removed because they were not the appropriate size for the hanging baskets required for the national flower show that came to Oldham in 2001. Rumours were spread that the Owl emblem was removed because the representation of a living creature is not allowed in Islam and so it was deemed offensive to Muslims. Now this appears to be a fairly sophisticated understanding of cultural difference, but this understanding did not lead to tolerance and harmony. Rather, it was used as a way of creating division. The lesson that can be drawn from this event is simply that understanding the diversity of ethnic groups and knowing of the diversity of cultural experiences does not necessarily lead to equality.

Conclusion

Diversity in the British population is taken for granted when it comes to a whole range of issues. Marketing companies divide the country into different segments for the purposes of selling to different types of customers. There are many references to the pink economy, the teenage market, the third age. Therefore, our concern should not simply be to acknowledge the existence of ethnic diversity but rather to try to understand the processes and mechanisms that lead to groups being marked out, and, as a result of that marking, subject to differential treatment, whether advantageous or disadvantageous. This process of marking is subject to change through time. It is not only the result of the activities of institutions and wider processes of governance, but is also in constant dialogical engagement with groups of people themselves.

A case study of this process is to be found in the civic disturbances of 2001. Police lore – the routines and customs that the police apply when dealing with people – marks certain groups for special treatment, in this case negative. This has an impact on how that group perceives itself in relation to the police and other groups involved in the same process. The nature of what we could call this ethnic group is not predetermined and does not have to exist forever. Changes in policy can result in different outcomes. Changes in police lore can ease tensions. The relationship with the police, then, is the beginning of a whole set of negative relations that lead to the disproportionate presence of blacks and Muslims in Britain's prisons. However, the statistical facts of this illustration of discrimination does not reveal the processes that led to one or other group being marked out for differential treatment. It is essential that local case studies are delineated.

The civil disturbances of 1981 were followed by the Scarman Report and a whole range of government programmes to deal with what were perceived as the 'problems' of the inner cities. A range of measures aimed at quelling discontent were put in place throughout the 1980s. The events of 2001 came two years after the Macpherson Report, and the rioting took place in areas that had been in receipt of numerous regeneration initiatives. It can also be argued that many more reports have been produced about these disturbances, but it remains apparent that some of the key questions about the relationship of the police and Asian Muslim young men remain beyond the serious questioning of public policy.

Notes

[1] This title is a modification of Michael Keith's (1993) seminal work *Race, riots and policing: Police lore and disorder in a multi-racist society*, London: UCL Press.

[2] For a useful summary and a large and comprehensive bibliography, see Bowling and Phillips (2002).

[3] Indeed, the House of Lords overturned some of the sentences received by the 'rioters' (30 January 2003) but did not accept the principle of mitigating circumstances that many had argued were important.

[4] Interestingly, the subsequent trials of young Asian men in Preston for the Burnley disturbances revealed a complete lack of ability by the Burnley police to handle the situation. This was glossed over by the inquiry as the police were one of the main commissioning bodies.

References

Abbot, D. (2002) 'Teachers are failing black boys', *The Observer*, 6 January.

Acheson, D. (1998) *Independent inquiry into inequalities in health report*, London: The Stationery Office.

Afshar, H. (1994) 'Muslim women in West Yorkshire: growing up with real and imaginary values amidst conflicting views of self and society', in H. Afshar and M. Maynard (eds) *The dynamics of race and gender: Some feminist interventions*, London: Taylor and Francis Ltd.

Ahmad, F., Modood, T. and Lissenburgh, S. (2003) *South Asian women and employment in Britain: The interaction of gender and ethnicity*, London: Policy Studies Institute.

Ahmad, W.I.U. (1992) 'The maligned healer: the "hakim" and western medicine', *New Community*, vol 18, no 4, pp 521-36.

Ahmad, W.I.U. (ed) (1993) *'Race' and health in contemporary Britain*, Buckingham: Open University Press.

Ahmad, W.I.U. (1996) 'The trouble with culture', in D. Kelleher and S. Hillier (eds) *Researching cultural differences in health*, London: Routledge.

Ahmad, W.I.U., Kernohan, E.E.M. and Baker, M.R. (1989) 'Influence of ethnicity and unemployment on the perceived health of a sample of general practice attenders', *Community Medicine*, vol 11, no 2, pp 148-56.

Alexander, C. (2000) *The Asian gang: Ethnicity, identity, masculinity*, Oxford: Berg.

Alexander, J.M. and Mohanty, C.T. (eds) (1997) *Feminist genealogies, colonial legacies, democratic futures*, London: Routledge.

Allen, S., and Wolkowitz, C. (1987) *Homeworking: Myths and realities*, Basingstoke: Macmillan.

Anderson, E. (1994) 'The code of the streets', *The Atlantic Monthly* (www.theatlantic.com/politics/race/streets.htm).

Appiah, L. (2001) *Mentoring: School business links*, Briefing Paper, May, Runnymede Trust.

Badger, F., Atkin, K. and Griffiths, R. (1989) 'Why don't general practitioners refer their disabled Asian patients to district nurses?', *Health Trends*, vol 21, pp 31-2.

Balarajan, R. and Bulusu, L. (1990) 'Mortality among immigrants in England and Wales, 1979-83', in M. Britton (ed) *Mortality and geography: A review in the mid-1980s, England and Wales*, London: OPCS.

Ballard, R. (1999) 'Socio-economic and educational achievements of ethnic minorities', Unpublished paper submitted to the Commission on the Future of Multi-Ethnic Britain, London: The Runnymede Trust.

Ballard, R. and Kalra, V.S. (1994) *Ethnic dimensions of the 1991 Census: A preliminary report*, Manchester: Census Microdata Unit, University of Manchester.

Barrett, G.A. (1999) 'Overcoming the obstacles? Access to bank finance for African-Caribbean enterprise', *Journal of Ethnic and Migration Studies*, vol 25, no 2, pp 303-22.

Bartley, M., Montgomery, S., Cook, D. and Wadsworth, M. (1996) 'Health and work insecurity in young men', in D. Blane, E. Brunner and R. Wilkinson (eds) *Health and social organization*, London: Routledge.

Basit, T.N. (1997) *Eastern values, Western milieu: Identities and aspirations of adolescent British Muslim girls*, Aldershot: Ashgate.

Battle, R.M., Pathak, D., Humble, C.G., Key, C.R., Vanatta, P.R., Hill, R.B. and Anderson, R.E. (1987) 'Factors influencing discrepancies between premortem and postmortem diagnoses', *Journal of the American Medical Association*, vol 258, no 3, pp 339-44.

Begum, N. (1992) *Something to be proud of: The lives of Asian disabled people and carers in Waltham Forest*, London: Waltham Forest Race Relations Unit and Disability Unit.

Beishon, S. and Nazroo, J.Y. (1997) *Coronary heart disease: Contrasting the health beliefs and behaviours of South Asian communities in the UK*, London: Health Education Authority.

Ben-Shlomo, Y., White, I.R. and Marmot, M. (1996) 'Does the variation in the socioeconomic characteristics of an area affect mortality', *British Medical Journal*, vol 312, pp 1013-14.

Berrington, A. (1994) 'Marriage and family formation among white and ethnic minority populations in Britain', *Ethnic and Racial Studies*, vol 17, no 3, pp 517-46.

Berthoud, R. (1997) 'Income and standards of living', in T. Modood, R. Berthoud, J. Lakey, J. Nazroo, P. Smith, S. Virdee and S. Beishon (eds) *Ethnic minorities in Britain*, London: Policy Studies Institute.

Berthoud, R. (1998) *The incomes of ethnic minorities*, ISER Report 98-1, Colchester: Institute for Social and Economic Research, University of Essex.

Berthoud, R. (1999) *Young Caribbean men and the labour market: A comparison with other groups*, York: Joseph Rowntree Foundation.

Berthoud, R. (2000a) 'Ethnic employment penalties in Britain', *Journal of Ethnic and Migration Studies*, vol 26, no 3, pp 389-416.

Berthoud, R. (2000b) *Family formation in multi-cultural Britain: Three patterns of diversity*, Colchester: Institute for Social and Economic Research, University of Essex (www.iser.essex.ac.uk/pubs/workpaps/pdf/2000-34.pdf).

Berthoud, R. (2001) 'Teenage births to ethnic minority women', *Population Trends*, vol 104, pp 12-17.

Berthoud, R. and Beishon, S. (1997) 'People, families and households', in T. Modood and R. Berthoud (eds) *Ethnic minorities in Britain: Diversity and disadvantage*, London: Policy Studies Institute.

Berthoud, R., Taylor, M. and Burton, J. (with contributions from T. Modood, N. Buck and A. Booth) (2000) *Comparing the transition from school to work among young people from different ethnic groups: A feasibility study for the Department of Education and Employment*, Colchester: Institute for Social and Economic Research, University of Essex.

Bhachu, P (1990) 'Culture ethnicity and class among Punjabi Sikh women in 1990s Britain', *New Community*, vol 17, no 3, pp 401-12.

Bhavnani, R. (1994) *Black women in the labour market: A research review*, London: Equal Opportunities Commission.

Bhavnani, R. and Coyle, A. (2000) 'Black and minority ethnic female managers in the UK', in M. Davidson and R. Burke (eds) *Women in management: Current research issues. Volume II*, London: Sage Publications.

Bhopal, K. (1998) 'How gender and ethnicity intersect: the significance of education, employment and marital status', *Sociological Research Online*, vol 3, no 3 (www.socresonline.org.uk/socresonline/3/3/6.html).

Bhopal, R. (1997) 'Is research into ethnicity and health racist, unsound, or important science?', *British Medical Journal*, vol 314, pp 1751-6.

Birmingham City Council (1998) *Black and minority ethnic communities' access to outer city housing*, Birmingham: Birmingham City Council (Housing Department).

Bisset, L. and Huws, U. (nd) *Sweated labour: Homeworking in Britain today*, London: Low Pay Unit.

Blackaby, D.H., Leslie, D.G., Murphy, P.D. and O'Leary, N.C. (2002) 'White/ ethnic minority earnings and employment differentials in Britain: evidence from the LFS', *Oxford Economic Papers*, vol 54, pp 270-97.

BLMN (*Black Labour Market News*) (1998) 'The New Deal', *Black Labour Market News*, issue 1 (first quarter), pp 9-19.

Bloor, M.J., Robertson, C. and Samphier, M.L. (1989) 'Occupational status variations in disagreements on the diagnosis of cause of death', *Human Pathology*, vol 30, pp 144-8.

Bowes, A., Dar, N. and Sim, D. (1997a) 'Tenure preference and housing strategy: an exploration of Pakistani experiences', *Housing Studies*, vol 12, no 1, pp 63-84.

Bowes, A., Dar, N. and Sim, D. (1997b) 'Life histories in housing research: the case of Pakistanis in Glasgow', *Quality and Quantity*, vol 31, pp 109-25.

Bowes, A., Dar, N. and Sim, D. (1998) *'Too white, too rough, and too many problems': A study of Pakistani housing in Britain*, Housing Policy and Practice Unit Research Report No 3, Stirling: Department of Applied Social Science, University of Stirling.

Bowling, B. and Phillips, P (2002) *Racism, crime and justice*, Essex: Longman.

Bradley, H. (2001) *Handling double disadvantage: Minority ethnic women and trade unions*, London: Economic and Social Research Council (www.regard.ac.uk).

Brah, A. (1994) '"Race" and "culture" in the gendering of labour markets: South Asian young Muslim women and the labour market', in H. Afshar and M. Maynard (eds) *The dynamics of race and gender: Some feminist interventions*, London: Taylor and Francis Ltd.

Brah, A. (1996) *Cartographies of diaspora: Contesting identities*, London: Routledge.

Brah, A. and Minhas, R. (1985) 'Structural racism or cultural difference: schooling for Asian girls', in G. Wiener (ed) *Just a bunch of girls: Feminist approaches to schooling*, Milton Keynes: Open University Press.

Brown, C. (1984) *Black and white Britain: The third PSI survey*, Aldershot: Gower.

Brown, C. and Gay, P. (1985) *Racial discrimination: 17 years after the act,* London: Policy Studies Institute.

Brownill, S. and Drake, J. (1998) *Rich mix: Inclusive strategies for urban regeneration*, Bristol/York: The Policy Press/Joseph Rowntree Foundation.

Bryan, B., Dadzie, S. and Scafe, S. (1985) *Heart of the race: Black women's lives in Britain*, London: Virago.

Burnley Task Force (2001) *Burnley Task Force Report*, Burnley: Burnley Task Force.

Burrows, R. (1997) 'The social distribution of the experience of homelessness', in R. Burrows, N. Pleace and D. Quilgars (eds) *Homelessness and social policy*, London: Routledge, pp 50-68.

Cabinet Office (2000) *Minority ethnic issues in social exclusion and neighbourhood renewal: A guide to the work of the Social Exclusion Unit and the Policy Action Teams so far*, London: Crown Copyright.

Cabinet Office (2001) *Towards equality and diversity: Implementing the employment and race directive*, London: Cabinet Office.

Cabinet Office (2002) *Cabinet Office Diversity Website* (www.diversity-whatworks.gov.uk/race.htm).

Cabinet Office (2003) *Ethnic minorities and labour markets*, London: The Stationery Office (www.strategy.gov.uk)

Cantle, T. (2001) *Community cohesion: A report of the independent review team*, London: Home Office.

Carby, H.V. (1982) 'White women listen! Black feminism and the boundaries of sisterhood', in Centre for Contemporary Cultural Studies, *The empire strikes back: Race and racism in 70s Britain*, London: Hutchinson Press.

Carter, J. (1999) 'Ethnicity, gender and equality', in R. Barot, H. Bradley and S. Fenton (eds) *Ethnicity, gender and social change*, London: Macmillan.

Carter, J., Fenton, S. and Modood, T. (1999) *Ethnicity and employment in higher education*, London: Policy Studies Institute.

CAVA (Economic and Social Research Council Research Group for the Study of Care, Values and the Future of Welfare) (2000) www.leeds.ac.uk/cava

Centre for Contemporary Cultural Studies (1982) *The empire strikes back: Race and racism in 70s Britain*, London: Hutchinson Press.

Chahal, K. (1999a) 'The Stephen Lawrence inquiry report, racist harassment and racist incidents: changing definitions, clarifying meaning?', *Sociological Research Online*, vol 4, no 1 (March) (www.socresonline.org.uk/socresonline/4/lawrence/chahal.html.

Chahal, K. (1999b) *Minority ethnic homelessness in London: Findings from a rapid review*, Report for NHS Executive (London), Preston: Federation of Black Housing Organisations and University of Central Lancashire.

Chahal, K. and Julienne, L. (1999) *'We can't all be white!': Racist victimisation in the UK*, York: Joseph Rowntree Foundation.

Chahal, K. and Temple, B. (2000) *Older people from minority ethnic communities: A housing research review*, Report by the Federation of Black Housing Organisations (FBHO) commissioned by Anchor Trust and Manningham Housing Association, London: FBHO.

Chamba, R., Ahmad, W., Hirst, M., Lawton, D. and Beresford, B. (1999) *On the edge: Minority ethnic families caring for severely disabled child*, Bristol/York: The Policy Press/Joseph Rowntree Foundation.

Chamberlain, M. (1999) 'Brothers, sisters, uncles and aunts: a lateral perspective on Carribbean families', in E. Silva and C. Smart (eds) *The new family?*, London: Sage Publications.

Chamberlain, M., Goulbourne, H., Plaza, D. and Owen, D. (1995) 'Living arrangements, family structure and social change of Caribbeans in Britain', *Changing Britain*, vol 4, London: Economic and Social Research Council.

Clunis, A. (2002) 'Stop our failing children', *Voice*, 25 March, pp 20-1.

CMEB (Commission on Multi-Ethnic Britain) (2000) *The future of multi-ethnic Britain*, London: Profile Books.

Coleman, D. (1995) 'International migration: demographic and socioeconomic consequences in the United Kingdom and Europe', *International Migration Review*, vol 19, no 1, pp 155-206.

Coleman, D. and Salt, J. (eds) (1996) *Ethnicity in the 1991 Census. Volume One: Demographic characteristics of the ethnic minority populations*, London: The Stationery Office.

Colley, L. (1992) *Britons: Forging the nation 1707-1837*, New Haven, CT: Yale University Press.

Connolly, P. (1998) *Racism, gender identities and young children*, London: Routledge.

Crawley, H. (2001) *Refugees and gender: Law and process*, Bristol: Jordan Publishing.

CRE (Commission for Racial Equality) (1984) *Race and council housing in Hackney: Report of a formal investigation*, London: CRE.

CRE (1988) *Homelessness and discrimination: Report of a formal investigation into the London Borough of Tower Hamlets*, London: CRE.

CRE (1996) *We regret to inform you*, London: CRE.

CRE (2001) *Statutory code of practice on the duty to promote race equality*, Commission for Racial Equality (www.cre.gov.uk).

CRE (2002a) *Ethnic minority women: Fact sheet* (www.cre.gov.uk/facts).

CRE (2002b) *Criminal justice in England and Wales: Fact sheets* (www.cre.gov.uk/facts).

Crenshaw, K. (1993) 'Whose story is it anyway? Feminist and anti-racist appropriations of Anita Hill', in T. Morrison (ed) *Race-ing justice, en-gendering power: Essays on Anita Hill and Clarence Thomas and the construction of social reality*, London: Chatto and Windus.

Crenshaw, K. (2000) 'Race reform and retrenchment: transformation and legitimation in anti-discrimination law', in L. Back and J. Solomos (eds) *Theories of race and racism*, London: Routledge.

Cross, M. (1994) *Ethnic pluralism and racial inequality*, Utrecht: University of Utrecht.

Dale, A., Fieldhouse, E.A. and Kalra V.S. (2001) *Labour market prospects for Pakistani and Bangladeshi women* (www.regard.ac.uk).

Dale, A., Fieldhouse, E.A., Shaheen, N. and Kalra, V.S. (2002) 'Routes into education and employment for young Pakistani and Bangladeshi women in the UK', *Work, Employment and Society*, vol 16, no 1, pp 5-27.

Dandeker, C. and Mason, D. (2001) 'The British armed services and the participation of minority ethnic communities: from equal opportunities to diversity?', *Sociological Review*, vol 49, no 2, pp 219-33.

Daniel, W.W. (1968) *Racial discrimination in England*, Harmondsworth: Penguin.

Davey Smith, G., Shipley, M.J. and Rose, G. (1990) 'Magnitude and causes of socioeconomic differentials in mortality: further evidence from the Whitehall study', *Journal of Epidemiology and Community Health*, vol 44, pp 265-70.

Davies, J. and Lyle, S. (with A. Deacon, I. Law, L. Julienne and H. Kay) (1996) *Discounted voices: Homelessness amongst young black and minority ethnic people in England*, Sociology and Social Policy Research Working Paper 15, Leeds: University of Leeds.

Davis, S. and Cooke, V. (2002) *Why do black women organise? A comparative analysis of black women's voluntary sector organisations in Britain and their relationship to the state*, Joseph Rowntree Foundation, London: Policy Studies Institute.

Denham, L. (2001) *Building cohesive communities: A report of the ministerial group on public order and community cohesion,* London: Home Office.

Dhooge, Y. (1981) *Ethnic difference and industrial conflicts*, Working Paper on Ethnic Relations 13, Birmingham: Social Science Research Council Research Unit on Ethnic Relations.

Dobson, J. and McLaughlan, G. (2001) 'International migration to and from the United Kingdom, 1975-1999: consistency, change and implications for the labour market', *Population Trends*, vol 106, pp 29-38.

Dobson, J., Khoser, K., McLaughlan, G. and Salt, J. (2001) *International migration and the United Kingdom: Recent patterns and trends*, Research Development and Statistics Occasional Paper 75, London: Home Office.

Donovan, J. (1986) *We don't buy sickness, it just comes*, Aldershot: Gower.

Drew, D. (1995) *'Race', education and work: The statistics of inequality*, Aldershot: Avebury.

Drew, D., Gray, J. and Sime, N. (1992) *Against the odds: The education and labour market experiences of black young people*, England and Wales Youth Cohort Study, Report RandD 68, Sheffield: Employment Department, Sheffield University.

DTI (Department of Trade and Industry) (2002a) *Equality and diversity: Making it happen*, London: The Stationery Office (www.dti.gov.uk/DTI/pub6354/30k/10/02/NP).

DTI (2002b) *Equality and diversity: The way ahead*, London: The Stationery Office (www.dti.gov.uk/DTI/pub6351/30k/10/02/NP).

Eade, J., Vamplew, T. and Peach, C. (1996) 'The Bangladeshis: the encapsulated community', in C. Peach (ed) *Ethnicity in the 1991 Census. Vol Two: The ethnic minority populations of Great Britain*, London: The Stationery Office.

Edwards, R. (1994) 'Taking the initiative: the government, lone mothers and provision', *Critical Social Policy*, vol 39, pp 36-50.

Elkins, M. and Olagundoye, J. (2001) *The prison population in 2000: A statistical review*, London: Home Office.

El Saadawi, N. (1980) *The hidden face of Eve: Women in the Arab world*, London: Zed Books.

Engels, F. (1987) *The condition of the working class in England*, Harmondsworth: Penguin.

EOC (Equal Opportunities Commission) (2000a) *Women and men in Britain series*, Manchester: EOC (www.eoc.org.uk).

EOC (2000b) *A checklist for gender proofing research*, Manchester: EOC (www.eoc.org.uk).

Erens, B., Primatesta, P. and Prior, G. (2001) *Health survey for England 1999: The health of minority ethnic groups*, London: The Stationery Office.

Eversley, D. and Sukdeo, F. (1969) *The dependants of the coloured Commonwealth population of England and Wales*, London: Institute of Race Relations.

FCO (Foreign and Commonwealth Office) (2000) *'A choice by right': Working group on forced marriage* (www.fco.gov.uk).

Felstead, A. and Jewson, N. (1996) *Homeworkers in Britain*, London: The Stationery Office.

Felstead, A. and Jewson, N. (1999) *In work, at home*, London: Routledge.

Fenton, S., Hughes, A. and Hine, C. (1995) 'Self-assessed health, economic status and ethnic origin', *New Community*, vol 21, no 1, pp 55-68.

Ferguson, R.F. (2004: forthcoming) 'Why America's black-white school achievement gap persists', in G. Loury, T. Modood and S. Teles (eds) *Race, ethnicity and social mobility in the US and UK*, Cambridge: Cambridge University Press.

Fieldhouse, E. and Gould, M.I. (1998) 'Ethnic minority unemployment and local labour market conditions in Great Britain', *Environment and Planning A*, vol 30, pp 833-53.

Frean, A. (2003) 'Black Africans in Britain lead way in education', *The Times*, 8 May (www.timesonline.co.uk).

Fredman, D. (2002) *The future of equality in Britain*, Working paper Series No 5, Manchester: Equal Opportunities Commission.

Gidley, G., Harrison, M. and Robinson, D. (1999) *Housing black and minority ethnic people in Sheffield*, Sheffield: CRESR, Sheffield Hallam University.

Gill, F. (2002) 'The diverse experiences of black and minority ethnic women in relation to housing and social exclusion', in P. Somerville and A. Steele (eds) *'Race', housing and social exclusion*, London: Jessica Kingsley, pp 159-77.

Gillborn, D. (1990) *'Race', ethnicity and education*, London: Unwin Hyman.

Gillborn, D. (1998) 'Race and ethnicity in compulsory schooling', in T. Modood and T. Acland (eds) *Race and higher education*, London: Policy Studies Institute.

Gillborn, D. and Gipps, C. (1996) *Recent research on the achievements of ethnic minority pupils*, London: Office for Standards in Education.

Gillborn, D. and Mirza, H. (2000) *Educational inequality: Mapping race, class and gender. A synthesis of research evidence*, London: Office for Standards in Education.

Gillborn, D. and Youdell, D. (2000) *Rationing education: Policy, practice, reform and equity*, Buckingham: Open University Press

Gilliam, S.J., Jarman, B., White, P. and Law, R. (1989) 'Ethnic differences in consultation rates in urban general practice', *British Medical Journal*, vol 299, pp 953-7.

Gilroy, P. (1987) *There ain't no black in the Union Jack: The cultural politics of race and nation*, London: Hutchinson.

Gray, P., Elgar, J. and Bally, S. (1993) *Access to training and employment for Asian women in Coventry*, Economic Development Unit Research Paper, Coventry: Coventry City Council.

Gregory, J. (2002) 'Discrimination, equality and human rights: dilemmas and contradictions', *Middlesex Research Seminar*, May, London: Middlesex University.

Guardian, The (2001a) 'Quiet riot', *Guardian Women*, 12 August, pp 8-9.

Guardian, The (2001b) 'Lifting the veil', *Guardian G2*, 14 August, pp 98-9.

Gupta, S., De Belder, A. and O'Hughes, L. (1995) 'Avoiding premature coronary deaths in Asians in Britain: spend now on prevention or pay later for treatment', *British Medical Journal*, vol 311, pp 1035-6.

Hagell, A. and Shaw, C. (1996) *Opportunity and disadvantage at age 16*, London: Policy Studies Institute.

Hall, S., Critcher, C., Jefferson, T., Clarke, J. and Roberts, B. (1978) *Policing the crisis: Mugging, the state and law and order*, London: Macmillan.

Hammonds, E. (1997) 'Toward a genealogy of black female sexuality: the problematic of silence', in J.M. Alexander and C.T. Mohanty (eds) *Feminist genealogies, colonial legacies, democratic futures*, London: Routledge.

Harding, S. and Maxwell, R. (1997) 'Differences in mortality of migrants', in F. Drever and M. Whitehead (eds) *Health inequalities: Decennial supplement no 15*, London: The Stationery Office.

Harrison, M. (1999) 'Theorising homelessness and "race"', in P. Kennett and A. Marsh (eds) *Homelessness: Exploring the new terrain*, Bristol: The Policy Press, pp 101-21.

Harrison, M. (with C. Davis) (2001) *Housing, social policy and difference: Disability, ethnicity, gender and housing*, Bristol: The Policy Press.

Harrison, M. (with D. Phillips) (2003) *Housing and black and minority ethnic communities: A review of the evidence base*, London: Office of the Deputy Prime Minister.

Haw, K. (1998) *Educating Muslim girls: Shifting discourses*, Milton Keynes: Open University Press.

Heath, A. and McMahon, D. (2000) *Ethnic differences in the labour market: The role of education and social class origins*, Working Paper 2000-01, Oxford: Department of Sociology, Oxford University.

Heath, A. and Ridge, J. (1983) 'Social mobility of ethnic minorities', *Journal of Biosocial Science*, (Supplement), vol 8, pp 169-84.

Heath, A. and Yu, S. (2001) 'Explaining ethnic minority disadvantage', Paper prepared for a Cabinet Office Report *Ethnic minorities in the labour market*, London: Performance and Innovation Unit.

Henderson, J. and Karn, V. (1987) *Race, class and state housing: Inequality and the allocation of public housing in Britain*, Aldershot: Gower.

Hepple, B., Coussey, M. and Choudhury, T. (2000) *Equality a new framework: Report of the independent review of the enforcement of UK anti-discrimination legislation*, Oxford: Hart Publishing.

Hill Collins, P. (1998) *Fighting words: Black women and the search for justice*, Minneapolis: University of Minnesota Press.

Holdaway, S. and Barron, A. (1997) *Resigners? The experience of black and Asian police officers*, Basingstoke: Macmillan.

Home Office (1998) *Statistics on race and the criminal justice system*, London: Home Office.

Home Office (2000) *Statistics on race and the criminal justice system 2000: A Home Office publication under Section 95 of the Criminal Justice Act 1991*, London: Home Office.

Housing Corporation London (1999) *Black and minority ethnic housing strategy for London*, London: The Housing Corporation (London Region).

Howes, E. and Mullins, D. (1999) *Dwelling on difference: An analysis of 1991 Census data*, London: London Research Centre.

Hubbock, J. and Carter, S. (1980) *Half a chance? A report on job discrimination against young blacks in Nottingham*, London: Commission for Racial Equality.

Hull, G., Bell Scott, P. and Smith, B. (1982) *All the women are white, all the blacks are men, but some of us are brave: Black women's studies*, New York, NY: The Feminist Press.

Ifekwunigwe, J. (1999) *Scattered belongings: Cultural paradoxes of 'race', nation and gender*, London: Routledge.

Iganski, P. and Mason, D. (2002) *Ethnicity, equality of opportunity and the British National Health Service*, Aldershot: Ashgate.

Iganski, P. and Payne, G. (1996) 'Declining racial disadvantage in the British labour market', *Ethnic and Racial Studies*, vol 19, no 1, pp 113-34.

Iganski, P. and Payne, G. (1999) 'Socio-economic re-structuring and employment: the case of minority ethnic groups', *British Journal of Sociology*, vol 50, no 2, pp 195-216.

Iganski, P., Payne, G. and Roberts, J. (2001) 'Inclusion or exclusion: reflections on the evidence of declining racial disadvantage in the British labour market', *International Journal of Sociology and Social Policy*, vol 21, nos 4-6, pp 184-211.

James, S.A., Strogatz, D.S., Wing, S.B. and Ramsey, D.L. (1987) 'Socioeconomic status, John Henryism and hypertension in blacks and whites', *American Journal of Epidemiology*, vol 126, pp 664-73.

Jenkins, R. (1986) *Racism and recruitment*, Cambridge: Cambridge University Press.

Jenkins, R. (1997) *Rethinking ethnicity*, London: Sage Publications.

Jewson, N. (1990) 'Inner city riots', *Social Studies Review*, vol 5, no 5, pp 170-4.

Jewson, N., Mason, D., Waters, S. and Harvey, J. (1990) *Ethnic minorities and employment practice: A study of six employers*, Department for Education and Employment Research Paper 76, London: DfEE.

Johnson, M.R.D., Owen D. and Blackburn C. (2000) *Black and ethnic minority groups in England: The second health and lifestyles survey*, London: Health Education Authority.

Jones, T. (1993) *Britain's ethnic minorities*, London: Policy Studies Institute.

JRF (Joseph Rowntree Foundation) (1993a) 'Involving disabled people in assessment', *Social Care Research Findings*, Issue 31.

JRF (Joseph Rowntree Foundation) (1993b) 'Ageing with a disability', *Social Care Research Findings*, Issue 34.

Karlsen, S. and Nazroo, J.Y. (2002) 'The relationship between racial discrimination, social class and health among ethnic minority groups', *American Journal of Public Health*, vol 92, pp 624-31.

Karlsen, S., Nazroo, J.Y. and Stephenson, R. (2002) 'Ethnicity, environment and health: putting ethnic inequalities in health in their place', *Social Science and Medicine*, vol 55, no 9, pp 1647-61.

Karn, V. (1997) '"Ethnic penalties" and racial discrimination in education, employment and housing: conclusions and policy implications', in V. Karn (ed) *Ethnicity in the 1991 Census. Volume Four: Employment, education and housing among the ethnic minority populations of Britain*, London: The Stationery Office, pp 265-90.

Karn, V., Mian, S., Brown, M. and Dale, A. (1999) *Tradition, change and diversity: Understanding the housing needs of minority ethnic groups in Manchester*, Source Research 37, London: The Housing Corporation.

Kaufman, J.S., Cooper, R.S. and McGee, D.L. (1997) 'Socioeconomic status and health in blacks and whites: the problem of residual confounding and the resiliency of race', *Epidemiology*, vol 8, no 6, pp 621-8.

Kaufman, J.S., Long, A.E., Liao, Y., Cooper, R.S. and McGee, D.L. (1998) 'The relation between income and mortality in U.S. blacks and whites', *Epidemiology*, vol 9, no 2, pp 147-55.

Keith, M. (1993) *Race, riots and policing: Police lore and disorder in a multi-racist society*, London: UCL Press.

Kennedy, H. (1993) *Eve was framed: Women and British justice*, London: Virago.

Kidd, C. (1999) *British identities before nationalism: Ethnicity and nationhood in the Atlantic world, 1600-1800*, Cambridge: Cambridge University Press.

Kings Fund (2001) *Black and ethnic minority women and health*, Kings Fund Information and Library Service (www.kingsfund.org.uk/eLibrary/html/).

Krieger, N. (1990) 'Racial and gender discrimination: risk factors for high blood pressure?', *Social Science and Medicine*, vol 30, pp 1273-81.

Krieger, N. and Sidney, S. (1996) 'Racial discrimination and blood pressure: the CARDIA study of young black and white adults', *American Journal of Public Health*, vol 86, no 10, pp 1370-8.

Krieger, N. Rowley, D.L., Herman, A.A., Avery, B. and Philips, M.T. (1993) 'Racism, sexism and social classs: implications for studies of health, disease and wellbeing', *Americal Journal of Preventive Medicine*, vol 9, supplement 2, pp 82-122.

Kundnani, A. (2001a) 'The summer of rebellion: special report', in *Campaign against Racism and Fascism 63*, August-September (www.carf.demon.co.uk/feat54.html).

Kundnani, A. (2001b) 'From Oldham to Bradford: the violence of the violated', *Race and Class*, vol 43, no 2, pp 105-10.

Law, I. (1996) *Racism, ethnicity and social policy*, London: Prentice Hall/Harvester Wheatsheaf.

Law, I., Davies, J., Phillips, D. and Harrison, M. (1996) *Equity and difference: Racial and ethnic inequalities in housing needs and housing investment in Leeds*, 'Race' and Public Policy Research Unit, Leeds: School of Sociology and Social Policy, University of Leeds.

Leicester City Council (1990) *Earnings and ethnicity*, Leicester: Leicester City Council.

Lemos and Crane (nd) *Black and minority ethnic registered social landlords*, Sector Study 1, London: The Housing Corporation.

Leslie, D.G., Drinkwater, S.J. and O'Leary, N. (1998) 'Unemployment and earnings among Britain's ethnic minorities: some signs for optimism', *Journal of Ethnic and Migration Studies*, vol 24, pp 489-506.

Lewis, G. (2000) *Race, gender and social welfare: Encounters in a postcolonial society*, London: Polity Press.

Lieberson, S. (1980) *A piece of the pie: Blacks and white immigrants since 1880*, Berkeley, CA: University of California Press.

Lord Chancellor's Department (2002) 'Rising trend in numbers of women and people from ethnic minorities appointed as judges. New official figures', Press Release, 30 October (www.gnn.gov.uk/gnn/national.nsf).

Mac an Ghaill, M. (1988) *Young, gifted and black: Student–teacher relations in the schooling of black youth*, Buckingham: Open University Press.

Macintyre, S., Maciver, S. and Soomans, A. (1993) 'Area, class and health: should we be focusing on places or people?', *Journal of Social Policy*, vol 22, no 2, pp 213-34.

Macpherson, W. (1999) *The Stephen Lawrence Inquiry: Report of an inquiry by Sir William Macpherson of Cluny*, Cm 4262-I, London: Home Office.

McCormick, B. (1986) 'Evidence about the comparative earnings of Asian and West Indian workers in Britain', *Scottish Journal of Political Economy*, vol 33, no 2.

McCrone, D. and Kiely, R. (2000) 'Nationalism and citizenship', *Sociology*, vol 34, no 1, pp 19-34.

McKeigue, P., Marmot, M., Syndercombe Court, Y., Cottier, D., Rahman, S. and Riermersma, R. (1988) 'Diabetes, hyperinsulinaemia, and coronary risk factors in Bangladeshis in East London', *British Heart Journal*, vol 60, pp 390-6.

McNaught, A. (1988) *Race and health policy*, London: Croom Helm.

Marmot, M.G., Adelstein, A.M., Bulusu, L. and OPCS (Office for Population Censuses and Surveys) (1984) *Immigrant mortality in England and Wales 1970-78: Causes of death by country of birth*, London: HMSO.

Mason, D. (1994) 'On the dangers of disconnecting race and racism', *Sociology*, vol 28, no 4, pp 845-58.

Mason, D. (1996) 'Themes and issues in the teaching of race and ethnicity in sociology', *Ethnic and Racial Studies*, vol 19, no 4, pp 789-806.

Mason, D. (2000) *Race and ethnicity in modern Britain* (2nd edn), Oxford: Oxford University Press.

Matheson, J. and Pullinger, J. (eds) (1999) *Social trends 29*, London: The Stationery Office.

Maxwell, R. and Harding, S. (1998) 'Mortality of migrants from outside England and Wales by marital status', *Population Trends*, vol 91, pp 15-22.

Maynard, M. (1994) "Race', gender and the concept of difference', in H. Afshar and M. Maynard (eds) *The dynamics of race and gender: Some feminist interventions* London: Taylor and Francis Ltd.

Metcalf, H. and Forth, J. (2000) *The business benefits of race equality at work*, Research Report 177, London: DfEE.

Miles, R. (1989) *Racism*, London: Routledge.

Mirza, H.S. (1992) *Young, female and black*, London: Routledge.

Mirza, H.S. (1997a) 'Mapping a genealogy of black british feminism', in H.S. Mirza (ed) *Black British feminism*, London: Routledge.

Mirza, H.S. (1997b) 'Black women in education: a collective movement for social change', in H.S. Mirza (ed) *Black British feminism*, London: Routledge.

Mirza, H.S. (1998) 'Race, gender and IQ: the social consequences of a social scientific discourse', *Race, education and ethnicity*, vol 1, no 1, pp 109-26.

Mirza, H.S (1999a) 'Black women into leadership? Issues of gender blind racial equality post Macpherson' *The Source: Public Management Journal*, 2 July (www.thesourcepublishing.co.uk).

Mirza, H.S. (1999b) 'Black masculinities and schooling: a black feminist response', *British Journal of Sociology of Education*, vol 20, no 1, pp 137-47.

Mirza, H.S and Reay, D. (2000a) 'Spaces and places of black educational desire: rethinking black supplementary schools as a new social movement', *Sociology*, vol 34, no 3, pp 521-44.

Mirza, H.S and Reay, D. (2000b) 'Redefining citizenship: Black women educators and the third space', in M. Arnot and J. Dillabough (eds) *Challenging democracy: International perspectives on gender, education and citizenship*, London: Routledge Falmer.

Mirza, H.S. and Rollock, N. (2001) 'Research review on black and minority ethnic women', Paper presented at the Rowntree Research Seminar 'Reviewing research on Black and Minority Ethnic Communities', July, York.

Mirza, H.S. and Sheridan, A. (2003) *Multiple identity and access to health: The situation, experience and identity of black and minority ethnic women*, Manchester: Equal Opportunities Commission.

Modood, T. (1993) 'The number of ethnic minority students in British higher education', *Oxford Review of Education*, vol 19, no 2, pp 167-82.

Modood, T. (1997a) 'Qualifications and English language', in T. Modood, R. Berthoud, J. Lakey, J. Nazroo, P. Smith, S. Virdee and S. Beishon (eds) *Ethnic minorities in Britain: Diversity and disadvantage*, London: Policy Studies Institute.

Modood, T. (1997b) 'Employment', in T. Modood, R. Berthoud, J. Lakey, J. Nazroo, P. Smith, S. Virdee and S. Beishon (eds) *Ethnic minorities in Britain: Diversity and disadvantage*, London: Policy Studies Institute.

Modood, T. (1997c) 'Culture and Identity', in T. Modood, R. Berthoud, J. Lakey, J. Nazroo, P. Smith, S. Virdee and S. Beishon (eds) *Ethnic minorities in Britain: Diversity and disadvantage*, London: Policy Studies Institute.

Modood, T. (1998) 'Ethnic minorities and the drive for qualifications', in T. Modood and T. Acland (eds) *Race and higher education*, London: Policy Studies Institute.

Modood, T. and Acland, T. (eds) (1998) *Race and higher education*, London: Policy Studies Institute.

Modood, T., Berthoud, R. and Nazroo, J. (2002) "Race', racism and ethnicity: a response to Ken Smith', *Sociology*, vol 36, no 2, pp 410-27.

Modood, T., Berthoud, R., Lakey, J., Nazroo, J., Smith, P, Virdee, S. and Beishon, S. (eds) (1997) *Ethnic minorities in Britain: Diversity and disadvantage*, London: Policy Studies Institute.

Mohanty, C.T. (1997) 'Women workers and capitalist scripts: ideologies of domination, common interests, and the politics of solidarity', in J. M. Alexander and C.T. Mohanty (eds) *Feminist genealogies, colonial legacies, democratic features*, London: Routledge.

Mohanty, C.T. (2000) 'Under Western eyes: feminist scholarship and colonial discourses', in L. Back and J. Solomos (eds) *Theories of race and racism*, London: Routledge.

Morrison, T. (1993) (ed) *Race-ing justice, en-gendering power: Essays on Anita Hill and Clarence Thomas and the construction of social reality*, London: Chatto and Windus.

NACAB (National Association of Citizens' Advice Bureaux) (1984) *Unequal opportunities: CAB evidence on racial discrimination*, London: NACAB.

Nairn, T. (1981) *The break-up of Britain: Crisis and neo-nationalism* (2nd edn), London: New Left Books.

Nazroo, J.Y. (1997) *The health of Britain's ethnic minorities: Findings from a national survey*, London: Policy Studies Institute.

Nazroo, J.Y. (1998) 'Genetic, cultural or socio-economic vulnerability? Explaining ethnic inequalities in health', *Sociology of Health and Illness*, vol 20, no 5, pp 710-30.

Nazroo, J.Y. (2001a) *Ethnicity, class and health*, London: Policy Studies Institute.

Nazroo, J.Y. (2001b) 'South Asians and heart disease: an assessment of the importance of socioeconomic position', *Ethnicity and Disease*, vol 11, no 3, pp 401-11.

Nazroo, J.Y. (2002) 'The racialisation of ethnic inequalities in health', in D. Dorling and L. Simpson (eds) *Statistics in society*, London: Arnold.

Nesbitt, S. and Neary, D. (2001) *Ethnic minorities and their pension decisions: A qualitative study of Pakistani, Bangladeshi and white men in Oldham*, Findings, York: York Publishing Services/Joseph Rowntree Foundation.

Noon, M. (1993) 'Racial discrimination in speculative applications: evidence from the UK's top one hundred firms', *Human Resource Management Journal*, vol 3, no 4, pp 35-47.

Oldham Independent Review Panel (2001) *Oldham Independent Review Report* (www.oldhamir.org.uk/OIR%20report.pdf).

OPCS (Office of Population Censuses and Survey) Immigrant Statistics Unit (1976) 'Country of birth and colour 1971-4', *Population Trends*, vol 2, pp 2-8.

OPCS Immigrant Statistics Unit (1977) 'New Commonwealth and Pakistani population estimates', *Population Trends*, vol 9, pp 4-7.

Osler, A., Street, C., Lall, M. and Vincent, K. (2002) *Not a problem? Girls and school exclusion*, London: Joseph Rowntree Foundation/National Children's Bureau.

Ousely, H. (2001) *Community pride not prejudice: Making diversity work in Bradford*, Bradford: Bradford Vision.

Owen, C., Mortimore, P. and Phoenix, A. (1997) 'Higher educational qualifications', in V. Karn (ed) *Ethnicity in the 1991 Census. Vol Four: Employment, education and housing among ethnic minority populations of Britain*, London: The Stationery Office.

Owen, D.W. (1992) *Ethnic minorities in Great Britain: Settlement patterns*, National Ethnic Minority Data Archive (1991 Census Statistical Paper 1), Coventry: Centre for Research in Ethnic Relations, University of Warwick.

Owen, D.W. (1993) *Ethnic minorities in Britain: Economic characteristics*, National Ethnic Minority Data Archive (1991 Census Statistical Paper 3), Coventry: Centre for Research in Ethnic Relations, University of Warwick.

Owen, D.W. (1994) *Ethnic minority women and the labour market: Analysis of the 1991 Census*, Manchester: Equal Opportunities Commission.

Owem, D.W. (1995) *Ethnic minorities in Britain: Patterns of population change, 1981-1991*, National Ethnic Minority Data Archive, 1991 Census Statistical Paper 10, Coventry: Centre for Research in Ethnic Relations, Univeristy of Warwick.

Owen, D.W. (1997) 'Changing patterns of residential segregation by ethnic group in England and Wales, 1981-91', Paper presented to the European Urban and Regional Research Network 1997 European Conference 'Regional Futures', 20-23 September, Europa-Universitat Viadrina, Frankfurt-am-Oder.

Owen, D.W. (1999) 'Making local estimates of minority ethnic group populations', Paper presented to the Population Geography Research Group 'Forecasting Populations' at the Annual Conference of the Royal Geographical Society with the Institute of British Geographers, University of Leicester, 7 January.

Owen, D.W. and Green, A.E. (1992) 'Occupational change among ethnic groups in Great Britain', *New Community*, vol 19, no 1, pp 7-29.

Owen, D.W. and Green, A.E. (2000) 'Estimating commuting flows for minority ethnic groups in England and Wales', *Journal of Ethnic and Migration Studies*, vol 26, pp 581-608.

Owen, D.W., Green, A., Pitcher, J. and Maguire, M. (2000) *Minority ethnic participation and achievements in education, training and the labour market*, Department for Education and Employment Research Report 225, Nottingham: DfEE.

Parmar, P. (1982) 'Gender, race and class: Asian Women in resistance', in Centre for Contemporary Cultural Studies, *The empire strikes back: Race and racism in 70s Britain*, London: Hutchinson Press.

Patel, P. (1997) 'Third wave feminism and Black women's activism', in H.S. Mirza (ed) *Black British feminism*, London: Routledge.

Pathak, S. (2000) *Race research for the future: Ethnicity in education, training and the labour market*, Research Topic Paper, Nottingham: DfEE.

Patterson, S. (1963) *Dark strangers*, London: Tavistock Publications.

Paxman, J. (1999) *The English: A portrait of a people*, London: Penguin.

Peach, C. and Byron, M. (1993) 'Caribbean tenants in council housing: "race", class and gender', *New Community*, vol 19, no 3, pp 407-23.

Peach, C. and Byron, M. (1994) 'Council house sales, residualisation and Afro Caribbean tenants', *Journal of Social Policy*, vol 23, no 3, pp 363-83.

Peach, G.C.K. (ed) (1975) *Urban social segregation*, London: Longman.

Peach, G.C.K. (1996) 'Does Britain have ghettos?', *Transactions of the Institute of British Geographers (New Series)*, vol 21, pp 216-35.

Penn, R. and Scattergood, H. (1992) 'Ethnicity and career aspirations in contemporary Britain', *New Community*, vol 19, no 1, pp 75-98.

Phillips, D. (1986) *What price equality?*, Greater London Council Housing Research and Policy Report 9, London: Greater London Council.

Phillips, D. (1996) 'Appendix 2: an overview of the housing needs of black and minority ethnic households. Census analysis', in M. Harrison, A. Karmani, I. Law, D. Phillips and A. Ravetz *Black and minority ethnic housing associations: An evaluation of the Housing Corporation's black and minority ethnic housing association strategies*, London: The Housing Corporation, pp 50-65.

Phillips, D. (1997) 'The housing position of ethnic minority group home owners', in V. Karn (ed) *Ethnicity in the 1991 Census. Vol Four: Employment, education and housing among the ethnic minority populations of Britain*, London: The Stationery Office, pp 170-88.

Phillips, D. and Karn, V. (1992) 'Race and housing in a property owning democracy', *New Community*, vol 18, no 3, pp 355-69.

Phillips, D. and Unsworth, R. (2002) 'Widening locational choices for minority ethnic groups in the social rented sector', in P. Somerville and A. Steele (eds) *'Race', housing and social exclusion*, London: Jessica Kingsley, pp 77-93.

Phillips, T. (2002) 'The time has come for zero-tolerance', *The Mail on Sunday*, 3 February, p 26.

Phoenix, A. (1996) 'Social constructions of lone motherhood: a case of competing discourses', in E. Bortolia Silva (ed) *Good enough mothering?*, London: Routledge.

Phoenix, A. (2001) 'Research review: children, families and young people', Paper presented at the Joseph Rowntree Research Seminar 'Reviewing Research on black and minority ethnic communities', July, York.

Phoenix, A. and Owen, C. (1996) 'From miscegenation to hybridity: mixed parentage and mixed relationships in context', in J. Brannen and B. Bernstein (eds) *Children, research and policy*, London: Taylor and Francis.

Pilgrim, S., Fenton, S., Hughes, T., Hine, C. and Tibbs, N. (1993) *The Bristol black and ethnic minorities health survey report*, Bristol: University of Bristol.

Pilkington, A. (1999) 'Racism in schools and ethnic differentials in educational achievement: a brief comment on a recent debate', *British Journal of Sociology of Education*, vol 20, no 3, pp 411-17.

Pirani, M., Yolles, M. and Bassa, E. (1992) 'Ethnic pay differentials', *New Community*, vol 19, no 1, pp 31-42.

Platt, L. and Noble, M. (1999) *Race, place and poverty*, York: Joseph Rowntree Foundation.

Puwar, N. (2001) 'The racialised somatic norm and the senior civil service', *Sociology*, vol 35, no 3, pp 651-70.

Radia, K. (1996) *Ignored, silenced, neglected: Housing and mental health care needs of Asian people in the London Boroughs of Brent, Ealing, Harrow and Tower Hamlets*, York: Joseph Rowntree Foundation.

Rai, D. and Thiara, R. (1997) *Re-defining spaces: The needs of black women and children in refuge support services and black workers in women's aid*, Bristol: Women's Aid Federation of England.

Ram, M. (1992) 'Coping with racism: Asian employers in the inner city', *Work, Employment and Society*, vol 6, no 4, pp 601-18.

Rassool, N. (1997) 'Fractured or flexible identities? Life histories of "black" diasporic women in Britain', in H.S. Mirza (ed) *Black British feminism*, London: Routledge.

Ratcliffe, P. (ed) (1996a) *Ethnicity in the 1991 Census. Volume 3: Social geography and ethnicity in Britain – Geographical spread, spatial concentration and internal migration*, London: The Stationery Office.

Ratcliffe, P. (1996b) *'Race' and housing in Bradford*, Bradford: Bradford Housing Forum.

Ratcliffe, P.' (1997) '"Race", ethnicity and housing differentials in Britain', in V. Karn (ed) *Ethnicity in the 1991 Census. Vol Four: Employment, education and housing among the ethnic minority populations of Britain*, London: The Stationery Office, pp 130-46.

Ratcliffe, P. (with M. Harrison, R. Hogg, B. Line, D. Phillips and R. Tomlins, and with Action Plan by A. Power) (2001) *Breaking down the barriers: Improving Asian access to social rented housing*, Coventry: Chartered Institute of Housing, on behalf of Bradford MDC, Bradford Housing Forum, The Housing Corporation, and Federation of Black Housing Associations.

Ray, L., Smith, D. and Wastell, L. (1999) 'The Macpherson Report: A view from Greater Manchester', *Sociological Research Online*, vol 4, no 1 (www.socresonline.org.uk/socresonline/4/lawrence/ray-smith-wastell.html).

Reay, D. and Mirza, H. (1997) 'A genealogy of the margins: black British supplementary schools', *British Journal of Sociology of Education*, vol 18, no 4, pp 477-99.

Rees, P. and Phillips, D. (1996) 'Geographical spread: the national picture', in P. Ratcliffe (ed) *Ethnicity in the 1991 Census. Vol 3: Social geography and ethnicity in Britain – Geographical spread, spatial concentration and internal migration*, London: The Stationery Office.

Rees, T. (1992) *Women and the labour market*, London: Routledge.

Reynolds, T. (1997) '(Mis)representing the black (super)woman', in H.S. Mirza (ed) *Black British feminism*, London: Routledge.

Reynolds, T. (1999) 'Re constructing African Caribbean mothering in Britain', Unpublished PhD thesis, South Bank University.

Richardson, R. and Wood, A. (1999) *Inclusive schools, inclusive society: Race and identity on the agenda*, London: Trentham Books.

Robinson, D. (2002) 'Missing the target? Discrimination and exclusion in the allocation of social housing', in P. Somerville and A. Steele (eds) *'Race', housing and social exclusion*, London: Jessica Kingsley, pp 94-113.

Robinson, D., Iqbal, B. and Harrison, M. (2002) *A question of investment: From funding bids to black and minority ethnic housing opportunities*, London: The Housing Corporation.

Robinson, V. (1989) 'Economic restructuring and the black population', in D.T. Herbert and D.J. Smith (eds) *Social problems and the city: New perspectives*, Oxford: Oxford University Press.

Rolfe, H. and Anderson, T. (2002) *A firm choice: Law firms' preferences in the recruitment of trainee solicitors*, London: National Institute of Economic and Social Research (www.niesr.ac.uk/pubs/law.pdf).

Rudat, K. (1994) *Black and minority ethnic groups in England: Health and lifestyles*, London: Health Education Authority.

Runnymede Trust (2000) *The Parekh Report: Commission on the Future of Multi-ethnic Britain*, London: Profile Books.

Runnymede Trust and the Radical Statistics Race Group (1980) *Britain's black population* London: Heinemann.

Sahgal, G. and Yuval-Davis, N. (1992) *Refusing holy orders: Women and fundamentalism*, London: Virago.

Salt, J. (1996) 'Immigration and ethnic group', in D. Coleman and J. Salt (eds) *Ethnicity in the 1991 Census. Vol One: Demographic characteristics of the ethnic minority populations*, London: The Stationery Office, pp 124-50.

Sandhu, H. (1998) 'Home affront', *Housing Today*, 1 October, p 19.

Sarre, P., Phillips, D. and Skellington, R. (1989) *Ethnic minority housing: Explanations and policies*, Aldershot: Avebury.

Scarman, Lord (1981) *The Scarman Report*, London: Home Office.

Schuman, J. (1999) 'The ethnic minority populations of Great Britain – latest estimates', *Population Trends*, vol 96, pp 33-43.

SEU (Social Exclusion Unit) (1998) *Bringing Britain together: A national strategy for neighbourhood renewal*, Cmnd 4045, London: The Stationery Office.

Sewell, T. (1997) *Black masculinity and schooling: How black boys survive modern schooling*, Stoke on Trent, Trentham Books.

Shaukat, N., De Bono, D.P. and Cruickshank, J.K. (1993) 'Clinical features, risk factors and referral delay in British patients of Indian and European origin with angina', *British Medical Journal*, vol 307, pp 717-18.

Shaw, C. (1988) 'Components of growth in the ethnic minority population', *Population Trends*, vol 52, pp 26-30.

Sheldon, T.A. and Parker, H. (1992) 'Race and ethnicity in health research', *Journal of Public Health Medicine*, vol 14, no 2, pp 104-10.

Shiner, M. and Modood, T. (2002) 'Help or hindrance? Higher education and the route to ethnic equality', *British Journal of Sociology of Education*, vol 23, no 2, pp 209-30.

Simmonds, F. (1997) 'My body myself: how does a black woman do sociology', in H.S. Mirza (ed) *Black British feminism*, London: Routledge.

Simpson, A. (1981) *Stacking the decks: A study of race, inequality and council housing in Nottingham*, Nottingham: Nottingham and District Community Relations Council.

Sloggett, A. and Joshi, H. (1994) 'Higher mortality in deprived areas: community or personal disadvantage?', *British Medical Journal*, vol 309, pp 1470-4.

Smaje, C. (1995) 'Ethnic residential concentration and health: evidence for a positive effect?', *Policy & Politics*, vol 23, no 3, pp 251-69.

Smaje, C. (1996) 'The ethnic patterning of health: new directions for theory and research', *Sociology of Health and Illness*, vol 18, no 2, pp 139-71.

Smith, D.J. (1976) *The facts of racial disadvantage*, London: Political and Economic Planning.

Smith, D.J. (1977) *Racial disadvantage in Britain*, Harmondsworth: Penguin.

Smith, D.J. (1981) *Unemployment and racial minorities*, London: Policy Studies Institute.

Smith, M.G. (1986) 'Pluralism, race and ethnicity in selected African countries', in J. Rex and D. Mason (1986) *Theories of race and ethnic relations*, Cambridge: Cambridge University Press.

Sodhi, D., Johal, S., Britain, E. and Steele, A. (2001) *The diverse needs of black and minority ethnic communities: An annotated bibliography of housing and related needs studies*, Manchester: Ahmed Iqbal Ullah Race Relations Archive.

Solomos, J. (1989) *Race and racism in contemporary Britain*, London: Macmillan.

Somerville, P., Sodhi, D. and Steele, A. (2000) *A question of diversity: Black and minority ethnic staff in the RSL sector*, Source Research 43, London: The Housing Corporation.

Soni Raleigh, V. and Balarajan, R. (1992) 'Suicide and self-burning among Indians and West Indians in England and Wales', *British Journal of Psychiatry*, vol 161, pp 365-8.

Southall Black Sisters (1998) *Free Zoora Shah! Update Leaflet*, Middlesex: Southhall Black Sisters.

Spivak, C.G. (1988) 'Can the subaltern speak?', in C. Nelson and L. Grossberg (eds) *Marxism and the interpretation of culture*, London: Macmillan Education.

Stewart, J.A., Dundas, R., Howard, R.A., Rudd, A.G. and Woolfe, C.D.A. (1999) 'Ethnic differences in incidence of stroke: prospective study with stroke register', *British Medical Journal*, vol 318, pp 967-71.

Sudbury, J. (1998) *'Other kinds of dreams': Black women's organisations and the politics of transformation*, London: Routledge.

Taylor, P. (1992) *Ethnic group data for university entry*, Project Report for Committee of Vice-Chancellors and Principals Working Group on Ethnic Data, Warwick: University of Warwick.

Third, H., Wainwright, S. and Pawson, H. (1997) *Constraint and choice for minority ethnic home owners in Scotland*, Edinburgh: Scottish Homes.

Thorogood, N. (1989) 'Afro-Caribbean women's experience of the health service', *New Community*, vol 15, no 3, pp 319-34.

Tomlins, R. (1999) *Housing experiences of minority ethnic communities in Britain: An academic literature review and annotated bibliography*, Centre for Research in Ethnic Relations Bibliographies in Ethnic Relations 15, Coventry: University of Warwick.

Tomlins, R. (with T. Brown, J. Duncan, M. Harrison, M. Johnson, B. Line, D. Owen, D. Phillips and P. Ratcliffe) (2001) *A question of delivery: An evaluation of how RSLs meet the needs of black and minority ethnic communities*, Source Research 50, London: The Housing Corporation.

Townsend, P. and Davidson, N. (1982) *Inequalities in health (the Black Report)*, Harmondsworth: Penguin.

UN (United Nations) (2000) *Gender and racial discrimination*, Report of the Expert Group Meeting 'UN Division for the Advancement of Women', 21-24 November, Zargreb (submission by K. Crenshaw).

Virdee, S. (1995) *Racial violence and harassment*, London: Policy Studies Institute.

Virdee, S. (1997) 'Racial harassment', in T. Modood, R. Berthoud, J. Lakey, J. Nazroo, P. Smith, S. Virdee and S. Beishon (eds) *Ethnic minorities in Britain: Diversity and disadvantage*, London: Policy Studies Institute.

Virdee, S., Modood, T. and Newburn, T. (2000) 'Understanding racial harassment in school', Final Report to the Economic and Social Research Council (www.regard.ac.uk).

Walby, S. (1994) 'Is citizenship gendered?', *Sociology*, vol 28, no 2, pp 379-95.

Walker, C. (1977) 'Migration: the impact on the population', *Population Trends*, vol 9, pp 24-6.

Walter, I. (1999) 'The embodiment of difference: a study of the transgression and violence among young black and white women', Unpublished PhD thesis, South Bank University.

Walvin, J. (1984) *Passage to Britain: Immigration in British history and politics*, Harmondsworth: Penguin (in association with Belitha Press).

Ward, R. and Jenkins, R. (eds) (1984) *Ethnic communities in business*, Cambridge: Cambridge University Press.

Weekes, D. (1997) 'Understanding black female subjectivity', Unpublished PhD thesis, Nottingham Trent University.

Westwood, S. and Bhachu, P. (eds) (1988) *Enterprising women: Ethnicity, economy and gender relations*, London: Routledge.

WEU (Women and Equality Unit) (2002a) *Key facts: Minority ethnic women in the UK* (www.womenandequalityunit.gov.uk).

WEU (2002b) *Key indicators of women's position in Britain*, London: The Stationery Office (www.womenandequalityunit.gov.uk).

Wild, S. and McKeigue, P. (1997) 'Cross sectional analysis of mortality by country of birth in England and Wales', *British Medical Journal*, vol 314, pp 705-10.

WNC (Women's National Commission) (2000) *Future female: A 21st century gender perspective*, London: The Stationery Office (www.thewnc.org.uk).

Woollett, E.A., Nicolson, P. and Marshall, H. (1993) *An investigation of parenthood and parenting practices in a multi-ethnic setting* (www.regard.ac.uk).

Wrench, J. and Qureshi, T. (1996) *Higher horizons: A qualitative study of young men of Bangladeshi origin*, Research Study 30, London: DfEE.

Yuval-Davis, N. (1993) 'Gender and nation', *Ethnic and Racial Studies*, vol 16, no 4, pp 621-32.

Zappone, K.E. (2001) *Charting the equality agenda: A coherent framework for equality strategies in Ireland North and South*, Belfast/Dublin: Equality Commission for Northern Ireland and The Equality Authority.

Zhou, M. (1997) 'Social capital in Chinatown: the role of community-based organizations and families in the adaptation of the younger generation', in L. Weis and M.S. Seller (eds) *Beyond black and white: New voices, new faces in the United States schools*, Albany, NY: State University of New York Press, pp 181-206.

Zhou, M. (2004: forthcoming) 'Ethnicity as social capital: community-based institutions and embedded networks of social relations', in G. Loury, T. Modood and S. Teles (eds) *Race, ethnicity and social mobility in the US and UK*, Cambridge: Cambridge University Press.

Index

Note: the abbreviation BME refers to black and minority ethnic.

A

activism, by BME women, 130-1
African ethnic groups
    and criminal justice system, 140-1,
        142
    see also Black–African ethnic group
African Asian ethnic group
    occupational status, 74
    performance at school, 56
    qualifications, 53, 54, 55
African-Caribbean ethnic group
    and criminal justice system, 140-1,
        142
    employment, 76, 77, 81, 83
    geographical distribution, 43
    housing, 114, 116
    social class and education, 63
African-Caribbean women, 124
    education, 128, 129
    as educators, 130
    family stereotypes, 125
    health, 132
age of BME groups, 33 4
    and housing needs, 113-14
    and labour market participation, 71
    and occupational mobility, 79
    of suspects arrested, 144-5
Anderson, E., 64
army, women in, 127
arrest rates, 144-5
Asian ethnic groups
    and civil disturbances, 147, 149-50
    and criminal justice system, 140, 143,
        144-5
    employment discrimination, 81, 82-3
    housing needs, 112
    performance at school, 58, 59
    self-employment, 83
    see also African Asian ethnic group;
        Bangladeshi ethnic group;
    Indian ethnic group; Pakistani ethnic
        group; South Asian ethnic groups
Asian men, relations with police, 145,
    147, 148, 149
Asian women
    family stereotypes, 125
    health, 132
asylum seekers, 24, 25, 49, 133

B

Balarajan, R., 92
Bangladeshi ethnic group
    education, 53, 54, 55, 56, 61, 62, 63,
        64, 65
    employment, 70-1, 73, 74, 76, 83
    fertility rates, 28
    geographical distribution, 38, 43, 44
    household structure, 34, 37
    housing, 105, 107
    migration to UK, 24, 26
    mortality and morbidity, 29, 89
    poverty, 85-6, 108-9
    share of minority ethnic population,
        32
    socioeconomic position, 62, 63, 64, 97
Bangladeshi women, 124
    education, 128
    employment, 126
    share of BME population, 123
Begum, N., 112-13
Berthoud, R., 28, 79-80, 85-6
birth rates, 27-31
Black ethnic groups
    born in UK, 26
    geographical distribution, 37, 38, 41
    housing, 107
    self-employment, 83
    and Stop and Search incidents, 143
    see also African ethnic groups; African-
        Caribbean ethnic group;
    Black–African ethnic group; Black–
        Caribbean ethnic group;
    Caribbean ethnic group
black and minority ethnic women
    community participation and activism,
        130-1
    education, 54, 55-6, 60, 62, 128-30
    employment, 71, 75, 83, 84, 85, 126-8
    family, 124-6
    health, 132
    housing needs, 114-15
    invisible in research and policy, 4-5,
        121-2, 134-5
    and law, 133, 141
    multiple identities, 123-4
    recognition of, 135
    representation, 134

demographic characteristics of BME
  groups
  age structure, 33-4
  ethnic structure, 31-3
  evolution of population, 21-3
  fertility and mortality, 27-31, 88-91,
    93-4, 95
  geographical distribution, 30-1, 37-48
  growth and change, 50-1
  household structure, 34-7
  and international migration, 23-7
  projected trends, 46, 48-50
Denham Report, 147-8
difference within difference, 106
disability, 112-13
discrimination *see* racial discrimination
domestic violence, 126

E

earnings, 77, 78
  see also household income
educational participation
  further education, 58-9, 130
  higher education, 59-62, 130
  women as educators, 130
educational performance
  of BME women, 128-9
  causes of ethnic difference, 62-5
  ethnic difference at school, 56-9
  polarities, 65-6
educational qualifications
  and employment, 80
  ethnic differences, 53-6, 63
  gender differences, 54, 55-6
  reliance on, 65
elders, housing needs of, 113-14
emigrants, 24
employment
  of BME women, 71, 75, 83, 84, 85,
    126-8
  explaining ethnic disadvantage in,
    79-83
  homeworking, 85
  participation, 70-3
  research and policy, 2
  self-employment, 83-4
  and settlement patterns, 70, 76
  see also household income;
    occupational mobility; occupational
    sectors; occupational status;
    unemployment
English identity, 18

EOC (Equal Opportunities
    Commission), 135
ethnic diversity
  awareness of, 9-10
  in Britain, 16-18
  and citizenship, 18
  measurement of, 13-16
ethnic marking, 139-40, 151
'ethnic minorities'
  designation of, 11-13
  see also minority ethnic groups
ethnic penalties, and housing, 106-7,
    111
ethnicity
  British conceptions of, 12-13
  concepts of race and, 10-11, 91-3

F

families
  of BME women, 124-6
  and self-employment, 84
family structure, 34-7, 84, 108, 125-6
fertility rates, 27-31
further education, 58-9, 130

G

Gay, P., 81
GCSE level qualifications, 54
gender
  and education, 62
  Caribbean boys at school, 57
  higher education, 60, 130
  qualifications, 54, 55-6
  and housing needs, 114-15
  and occupational status, 75, 127-8
  and prison population, 133, 141
  and self-employment, 83, 84
  structure of BME groups, 32, 123
  see also black and minority ethnic
    women
gender research, invisibility of BME
    women in, 135
genetic explanations of health
    inequalities, 91-3, 132
geographical distribution, 25, 37-48, 51
  of births in Britain, 30-1
  and employment, 70, 73, 76
  and health inequalities, 102
  residential relocation, 117-19
geographical segregation, 41-8
  see also residential segregation
ghettoisation, 110
Gray, P., 82

U
unemployment, 71-3, 79, 97, 127
Unsworth, R., 118
urban disturbances *see* civil disturbances

V
victim blaming, 2-3
vocational qualifications, 55, 56

W
West Midlands, BME population in,
   37-8
White ethnic groups, and Stop and
   Search, 143
white youths, and Oldham disturbances,
   149-50
women *see* black and minority ethnic
   women
Women's National Commission, 135

Y
youth culture, of Caribbean boys, 57

Z
Zarb, G., 113
Zhou, M., 64

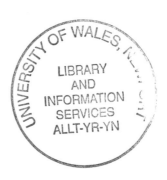